THE PRACTICE OF VETERINARY DENTISTRY

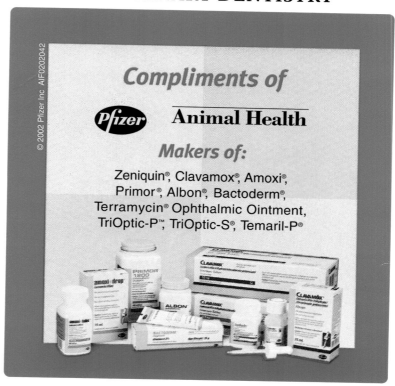

Compliments of

Pfizer **Animal Health**

Makers of:

Zeniquin®, Clavamox®, Amoxi®,
Primor®, Albon®, Bactoderm®,
Terramycin® Ophthalmic Ointment,
TriOptic-P™, TriOptic-S®, Temaril-P®

THE PRACTICE OF
VETERINARY DENTISTRY
A *Team* Effort

JAN BELLOWS, DVM

IOWA STATE UNIVERSITY PRESS / AMES

Jan Bellows, DVM, received his doctor of veterinary medicine degree from Auburn School of Veterinary Medicine. Dr. Bellows is a diplomate of both the American Board of Veterinary Practitioners and the American Veterinary Dental College and a fellow of the Academy of Veterinary Dentistry. Additionally, Dr. Bellows is an assistant clinical professor in the Department of Oral Medicine at Nova University School of Dentistry. He has been the owner/operator of The Pet Health Care Center in Pembroke Pines, Florida, for over 20 years.

© 1999 Iowa State University Press, Ames, Iowa 50014
All rights reserved

Iowa State University Press
2121 South State Avenue, Ames, Iowa 50014

ORDERS: 1-800-862-6657
OFFICE: 1-515-292-0140
FAX: 1-515-292-3348
WEB SITE: www.isupress.edu

∞ Printed on acid-free paper in the United States of America

First edition, 1999

Library of Congress Cataloging-in-Publication Data
  Bellows, Jan
  The practice of veterinary dentistry: a team effort
  Jan Bellows. — 1st ed.
  p. cm.
  Includes bibliographical references (p.   ) and index.
  ISBN 0-8138-2617-9 (alk. paper)
  1. Veterinary dentistry.   I. Title.
  SF867.B45   1999
  636.089′76—dc21

The last digit is the print number: 9 8 7 6 5 4 3 2 1

➣ Gerry Selin is a true friend of those striving to do well. I dedicate this book to him.

LETTER OF APPRECIATION

Dear Dr. Bellows,

There are not words to express the gratitude this family feels towards you for the remarkable work you have done in saving our "Harley."

When we were referred to you, I felt hopeful that Harley's terrible mouth condition would be improved, but I never thought that I would see the radical changes I have witnessed. Underweight, in pain, and with other physical ailments, to see our Harley now would make you think we had a new dog. And, indeed, in some ways we do!

On Thursday, May 21st, Harley had 15 teeth removed (all he had left). We took him "home" that night. The next morning he had a checkup and we headed back to North Florida where we live. Eating and drinking nothing on Friday and Saturday, you suggested trying him on his favorite things first. On Sunday, he had a drink from the swimming pool (his favorite water), then some cooked chicken (his favorite food). That evening, he was eating dry kibble from our other dogs' dishes, enthusiastically! And with this, every day has been better and better.

Regaining strength rapidly, eating on his own (I had hand fed him for about a year), all odor and drooling completely gone, Harley in a week was running and playing with his mates—Nitti, a poodle, and Bella, a large shepard [sic] mix. Then on Memorial Day, May 31st, he got his bark back— he had not barked in several years. Three weeks after surgery, he has put on 3 pounds, runs and plays like he did when he was a puppy, and has returned to all his endearing old habits, including carrying around his favorite squeeker toy (also not done in years). His mouth has completely healed and he doesn't seem to know he has no teeth. Even the side effects of a previous illness are completely gone.

We cannot thank you enough for what you have done for Harley and this family. He is our most cherished "child," and so you have given us all new life and joy.

With gratitude
Mullie Hack & Harley

❧CONTENTS

✦FOREWORD BY GERARD B. SELIN

I have been associated with the veterinary profession for more than 40 years. During this time I have been instrumental in introducing a number of modalities that were innovative at the time but have become important daily necessities in the life of every practice. These included such diverse areas as inhalation anesthesia, heartworm testing, allergy testing and treatment, cardiac medication, improved methods for diagnosing internal parasitism, and, most recently, veterinary dentistry. Each of these proved a challenge because there was a large group of academics and practitioners who felt that these new techniques were not needed and the status quo was just fine. It is hard to believe that as recently as 1971 most practitioners believed that heartworm disease occurred in a small portion of the country and was not worthy of consideration as a major threat to health outside of this area. In fact, the pharmaceutical company that developed diethylcarbamazine, the only drug that prevented the disease at the time, did not even have a heartworm claim on its label. It was marketed for use against roundworms. According to sales figures published at the time, less than 1 million dollars worth of the product was used. Compare that with the universal testing that is now being done for heartworm disease and the sales of well over 100 million dollars worth of preventive products. This is reflected in healthier animals, happier clients, and vastly increased revenues for practices throughout the land.

Why discuss the heartworm story in a book about veterinary dentistry? Because it was not until veterinarians became convinced that there was danger to their patients from this dreaded disease and therefore integrated it into their regular preventive program that it become meaningful.

And so it is with dentistry. Oral disease, in its many forms, represents a major threat to all species of companion animals. Recent studies show that all age groups are at risk. Unless practitioners are consistent about examining every animal that enters their clinic for the existence of oral disease, they are not practicing quality medicine. Oral disease can not only be a source of pain to the animal but can be the pathway to life-threatening systemic disorders that affect the liver, kidneys, and heart. Over the past 10 years, articles have appeared in leading journals attesting to the relationship of dental disease to overall health.

It is difficult to understand why, after 15 years of exposure to thousands of hours of continuing education, hundreds of articles, more than 12 texts, and the creation of the Academy of Veterinary Dentistry and the American Veterinary Dental College, many veterinarians refuse to make veterinary dentistry an integral part of their practices. I have been told by the owners of successful multiveterinarian practices that include people board certified in internal medicine and surgery that they do not choose to include dentistry in their practices. This is like arbitrarily saying they will not treat diseases of the eye. Why is pain and infection in the oral cavity any less worthy of treatment than pain and infection in any other part of the body? Where is the client to go for help? Not only are these practitioners shortchanging their patients and clients but they are being fiscally irresponsible toward their practices. An interesting analogy can be drawn from the field of equine medicine. For decades a number of equine practitioners turned their backs on floating teeth. Laypeople experienced with caring for horses became proficient in the technique and became known to many horse owners as "horse dentists." They were filling a need that was being neglected by the veterinary profession, and it did not appear to infringe on any practice laws. Recently, there has been a great deal of interest on the part of equine practitioners to regain this aspect of their practices.

The difference between floating horse teeth and performing a prophy on small animals, which has kept the latter out of lay hands, is that general anesthesia is not required in the case of the equine procedure. However, having said that, there was the case in California in the late 1980s in which the veterinary association sought relief from the legislature to keep groomers from scaling dogs' teeth.

As the secretary/treasurer of the American Society of Veterinary Dental Technicians (ASVDT), I am in contact with thousands of veterinarians and technicians throughout the country. I have firsthand knowledge of the dramatic increase in revenues of practices that have made dentistry an integral part of their practices. Many have quoted 20 to 30 percent gains with the same client base! In some cases this has amounted to hundreds of thousands of dollars, and these are not dental referral practices.

I have also received hundreds of calls and letters from technicians and assistants who perform dental prophys. They relate their frustrations with employers who refuse to stress the importance of routine prophylaxes. The technician is the core of a dental practice just as the dental hygienist is in human dentistry. Properly trained, technicians are a profit center that does not require the intervention of the veterinarian. They can be the dental liaison with the client about proper home care and telephone follow-up. In practices where this procedure is followed, the clients have responded favorably to the attention and care their animals are receiving, which further bonds those clients to the practices.

The telephone number of the ASVDT is listed in our local phone book, which has led to many interesting phone calls from clients in Sarasota County, Florida. Because they see "dental" in our title, they think we perform dental procedures. When informed that we do not, they ask where they can go to get their animals' dental problems taken care of. We tell them to contact their regular veterinarian, and often they tell us that their veterinarian has either told them that the animal does not need treatment or has displayed such a lack of knowledge that they want more competent help. There is a board-certified dentist about 70 miles away, and in most cases, they are happy to make the trip to gain relief for their pets. I know most of the practitioners that are involved, and they have always argued with me that their clients will not pay for dental services. The same client spends four hours on the road and pays a specialist's fees.

Dr. Bellows is an outstanding example of how dentistry can grow a practice exponentially and gain extraordinary loyalty from clients. He is the exception, in that he is board certified in dentistry and has a referral practice in addition to his general practice. Over the past few years, I have spent a number of days observing his practice and speaking to his clients.

His client base covers the entire financial spectrum, from retirees living on meager pensions to well-to-do professionals. Each of his clients receives the same information about the great need for regular dental examinations and prophylaxes. If a problem area is discovered, he will take a Polaroid close-up that clearly (and dramatically) shows the condition. This not only helps the client in the exam room understand the situation but gives the client something to take home to family members that clearly demonstrates the need for treatment.

Dr. Bellows also uses the primary dental diagnostic tool, a dental X-ray unit, to great advantage. When an animal is under anesthesia for a teeth cleaning, and there is the slightest indication of subgingival problems, a series of X rays are taken. If they are indicative of a condition that requires treatment, the radiographs are enlarged by placing them in a compact (and inexpensive) unit that allows the client to see the pathology. All clients express their pleasure that X rays are included in the diagnostic process. As each of these steps take place, they are circled on a printed fee schedule so clients know exactly what they are being charged and *why* they are being charged. In all of my visits, I never saw a client refuse suggested treatments. When I spoke to them privately, they all felt that they were being treated fairly and (most important of all) their pets were receiving the best possible care.

A dental X-ray unit is essential to the practice of veterinary dentistry. Without it you are working in the dark. It is also the wisest investment you can make. Used properly, it will pay for itself in four to six months. Contrast this to the big 300ma machines that take years to pay for. If you are going to rely on your large machine for dentistry, you will only use it a fraction of the time because of the inconvenience of bringing an animal to the X-ray room. The results obtained by using a portion of a large cassette are so poor, in most cases, that a proper diagnosis cannot be reached. The dental X ray is like a simple point-and-shoot camera that produces clear and well-defined radiographs.

In my discussions with veterinarians throughout the country, it is heartening to find a growing number recognizing the importance of including dentistry in the mainstream of their practices. This has been borne out by their supporting continuing education programs for members of their staffs as well as schooling themselves in advanced dental techniques. Unfortunately, they represent a small percentage of the 20,000 plus practices that care for our small animal population. Veterinary medicine will not attain its finest hour until all practices are treating the whole animal.

Those of us who are passionate about the advance of veterinary dentistry have much to thank Jan Bellows for. He spent hundreds of hours creating the home study course for the ASVDT that has been purchased by over 2200 technicians and veterinarians. Now he has written this very practical book about how to develop your veterinary dental practice. Put his suggestions to work. I've seen the great results.

❧PREFACE

The Practice of Veterinary Dentistry: A Team Effort was conceived from a need to inform and educate, a real need to serve veterinarians, their staff, the public, and most importantly companion animals. For the major part of the 25 years I have been actively involved in veterinary medicine, small animal dentistry has been in its infancy. Most practitioners have poorly understood veterinary dentistry and its importance to the overall health of their patients. Dentistry has never been accepted as a medical modality; it has been pushed into the background. For over 95 percent of veterinarians, the practice of veterinary dentistry means removing calculus from crowns and extracting mobile teeth. The time has come to learn how to conduct a meaningful veterinary dental practice, conforming to present knowledge.

It is not that veterinarians do not want to practice quality dentistry; it is that most cannot determine how

- To understand dental principles that unfortunately were not taught in school
- To acquire and use the proper equipment
- To perform or refer endodontics, periodontal surgery, and orthodontics
- To train staff to care for dental patients and clients
- To convince owners of the importance of dentistry to overall health
- To integrate dentistry into their general practice

These are the goals of this book. It is written from my "on-the-job-training" experience. In 1984 I attended a veterinary dental wet lab given by Dr. Keith Grove in Vero Beach, Florida. He has degrees in veterinary medicine and human dentistry. I came back to my practice convinced I had to increase my expertise and knowledge of veterinary dentistry to properly care for my patients and clients. I knew this was important for me to do but was not sure how to do it.

The first hurdle was understanding new words. There were hundreds that I had little clue to their meanings. Some examples: *furcations, anterior crossbite, college tipped pliers, edgewise appliance, mesial, light-cured bonding, labial, pocket, Gracey curette,* and *gutta-percha.* At the time there were only three recognized texts on veterinary dentistry. Reading them did help, but I had problems tying the concepts to practicing the art.

The next hurdle was working with dental equipment. For this I thank my dentist, Dr. Andrew Stutz. Andy would come over any time I had questions on how to take radiographs, work with materials, and make therapy decisions based on pathology presentation. Equipping my dental practice meant trying to determine what to buy, who to buy from, and how to use the equipment. I soon learned that purchasing used radiographic machines was not the way to go. Both used machines I acquired lasted six months. The new one I purchased eight years ago is still giving excellent service.

I still needed more knowledge so I could be confident enough to practice veterinary dentistry and convince clients to let me take care of observed pathology. I thank Dr. Tom Mulligan for his contagious enthusiasm, Pete Emily, Colin Harvey, Gary Beard, Ben Colmery, Steve Holmstrom, Ed Eisner, Pat Frost, Chuck Williams, Suzie Aller, James Anthony, Gary Goldstein, Keith Grove, Don Ross (for my first formal exposure to veterinary dentistry in 1972), Sandra Manfra-Marretta, Chris Visser, and Bob Wiggs for their contribution to veterinary dentistry and to my education. Their selfless dedication to sharing is appreciated. I especially thank veterinary dentists Paul Cleland, Steve Holstrom, and Ken Lyon; human dentists Larry Grayhills and Barry Staley; veterinarian Ron Stone; and my parents Marvin and Selma Bellows for reviewing the manuscript.

The learning process is continual. Hardly a day goes by that I do not learn a new way of doing my job better. On your journey toward creating the best dental practice, there will be questions. Any of the above dental experts are eager to help you.

Experts from industry have helped me throughout my journey. I thank Dave Harmsen and Rod Miers from Pharmacia & Upjohn Animal Health for their support of veterinary dentistry. Seeing the need to educate their sales teams and veterinarians in dental concepts, they have presented hundreds of seminars and published *The Smile Book.* This book, which I authored, helps veterinarians pictorially explain dental procedures to their clients.

I also thank Clint Harris, Marge Mc Donnell, Adrienne Silkowitz, and Keith Stuart from Henry Schein, Inc., for equipment support over the years. Henry Schein, Inc., has been at the forefront of veterinary dentistry for at least 30 years. Ken Bowman and Dr. Steve Lotz from VRX Pharmaceuticals have been there any time I need support for home care information.

I especially thank Gerry Selin for being the wind behind my dental journey and this book. I met Gerry at the American Animal Hospital Association meeting in San Francisco in 1990, where I gave my first major meeting presentation and Gerry was receiving an award for essentially bringing dentistry to veterinary medicine. We had never met before. My wife and I sat next to Gerry at the awards dinner. According to my wife, "everything happens for a reason." Our meeting led to a wonderful relationship based on his passion for pushing dentistry into the forefront of veterinary medicine. Gerry is a true visionary: he sees a need and figures out a selfless way to fill it. Before urging me to write this book, he created the American Society of Veterinary Dental Technicians, and as of this writing the society has over 2000 members. He was also the force behind converting my dental computer teaching program into a video format used to train and qualify veterinary dental technicians.

The Practice of Veterinary Dentistry: A Team Effort is divided into eight chapters. The book is not meant to cover every veterinary dental procedure performed, and it is not meant to show step-by-step how to perform procedures. Do not look for references in each chapter. This book is written for the veterinarians, technicians, and kennel persons who want to create a dental practice within their practices. You will be exposed to

- Veterinary dental philosophy
- Normal anatomy
- How to conduct an oral examination
- How to equip your practice
- How to take and interpret radiographs
- An explanation of the importance of the 12 steps of professional teeth cleaning
- How to plan dental therapy
- How to propose your recommendations to pet owners so that they will understand and accept needed therapy for their animals

A book of this scope could not have been produced without the willingness of the publisher to struggle with the revisions and the sometimes illegible handwriting. Gretchen Van Houten, editor-in-chief, and Lynne Bishop and Betsy Hovey, editors, were there every step of the journey. This book could not have been accomplished without the talents and assistance of these individuals.

Enjoy

THE PRACTICE OF
VETERINARY DENTISTRY

1. PHILOSOPHY AND TEAMWORK

What makes men great is their ability to decide what is important, and then focus their attention on it.
—ANONYMOUS

DENTAL PHILOSOPHY

Clients expect the veterinarian to do whatever has to be done to keep their animals healthy. They bring their pets to us for premium care. Pet owners trust us to do our best. What is the best when it comes to dentistry? By the time you finish reading this book, *best* will be the only way you practice small animal dentistry—there are no other choices.

Veterinarians have virtually neglected the oral cavity in the past. "Fire engine" dentistry, practiced only when the mouth is on fire, is not the best way to deliver premium health care. The veterinarian and staff must treat the oral cavity as professionally as they do other vital organs.

Unfortunately, as of this writing, veterinarians do not receive much dental education in veterinary school, so many feel it must not be important. The only attack most veterinarians mount against dental disease is removal of supragingival calculus once periodontal disease is established.

In the past the veterinarian was the lone player against dental disease. Dentistry was usually practiced on a hit-or-miss basis with no true game plan. After each prophy, disease retreated, going undercover beneath the gingiva and becoming a more powerful competitor by "eating away" the supporting bone around teeth. When the veterinarian removed calculus a year later, the disease had progressed, and teeth were often lost.

In dental offices for humans, teeth cleaning and polishing represent about 30 percent of caseload and income, with the remaining 70 percent related to care of oral pathology. The opposite is true in veterinary offices: roughly 70 percent of dentistry is devoted to cleaning teeth and 30 percent to extractions. With attention given to abnormalities noted in the oral exam and the active pursuit of therapy for existing oral pathology, the amount of the veterinary practice's periodontal, endodontic, and orthodontic care raises its therapy percentages, making them the equivalent of those of dental practices for humans.

In many small animal practices, dentistry accounts for less than 10 percent of gross income. When the proper dental program is put into effect, a dental practice is created that will provide an additional 40 percent in gross income. These are actual increases brought to my attention from veterinarians around the country.

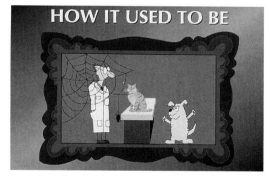

Fig. 1.1.

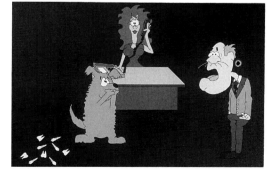

Fig. 1.2.

Philosophical Musts

- The veterinarian and staff have opportunities to recognize dental disease and recommend therapy. An oral examination *must* be part of every checkup regardless of what the animal is presented for. Just because a dog or cat may present with a broken leg, this does not mean that existing periodontal disease should not be cared for on the operating table.

- The need for dentistry *must* be integrated into your practice philosophy so that it becomes as routine as a vaccine program. Once or twice yearly, your client comes in expecting vaccinations to prevent disease; this is an opportunity for dental evaluation and care. As soon as the pet owners understand the need for regular dental exams and teeth cleaning, they are pleased to comply.

- The veterinarian and staff *must* educate clients about the need for dentistry and convince them of its importance. Based on statistics, 25 percent of your clients will accept whatever you say immediately; another 60 percent will take a little time to embrace your recommendations, dental or otherwise; the remaining 15 percent will not accept your recommendations and may be happier at a practice that does not stress quality care.

- The goal of a veterinary dental practice *must* be to provide the quality of care that is provided for every other part of the animal's body. To achieve this goal, you *must* commit to developing clinical skills and working with adequately trained and dedicated staff.

- Small animal dentistry *must* be done at the same level of perfection that you demand for all other modalities. Removing the calculus from the surface of an animal's teeth and ignoring disease below the gingiva is not practicing quality medicine. By probing and taking dental radiographs, you can determine what problems exist.

- Dentistry *must not* be practiced on a superficial basis. The mouth must be examined in depth. Scheduling an excessive number of professional teeth cleanings each day restricts in-depth examinations and therapy for disclosed lesions, which creates a lose, lose, lose situation.

  — The patient loses when the veterinarian does not treat oral pathology because of a lack of knowledge, interest, or time.

  — The client loses if the pet does not receive the best care.

  — The practice loses by missing income from not treating dental pathology.

- The veterinarian and technician *must* have knowledge and appreciation for normal dog and cat oral anatomy. You *must* examine every patient's mouth on each visit.

- Soon it becomes second nature to recognize oral abnormalities. But identifying oral problems is only part of the challenge. You must also formulate a treatment plan and personally convey the urgency of treatment to the owner.

- Veterinarians *must* believe in the importance of dentistry to every patient. If you do not fully believe in providing the best dental care, the job cannot be done—staff will not promote dentistry, and clients will not get the message. By accepting the importance of dentistry for every patient, you will be able to add a whole new dimension of health care and to increase the revenue stream to your practice.

Dental Disease Is Progressive

- When you observe a dental problem at any stage of its development, it *must* be brought to the client's attention, and you *must* advise immediate treatment to keep it from progressing. Lesions will worsen with neglect. We know that bacteria, when left untreated, will multiply, producing by-products that destroy supporting bone, which progresses to untreatable dental disease and multiple organ failure.

- In an exam room setting, each time you observe grade one gingivitis apical to the maxillary fourth premolar crown, you *must* convince your client to allow an immediate professional teeth cleaning. Gingivitis is an inflammation of the gingiva caused by bacteria. Failure to deliver therapy will lead to progressive disease.

- Every member of your staff *must* be a part of the dental team because dentistry begins with the phone call answered by the receptionist. The technician then meets your client in the exam room and has an opportunity to speak about dental care. The kennel person handles the pet before and after surgery. The veterinarian then diagnoses and treats the dental problems. Finally, the owner must provide home care.

No other veterinary modality benefits so much from having a backup team that can discern the stages of disease. Developing this team takes effort and direction from the team captain—the veterinarian.

- The veterinarian *must* schedule more time for oral examination and therapy, or the result will be that patient dental needs are not treated (Fig. 1.3).

- Where is the time going to come from? With the responsibilities of managing staff, clients, suppliers, and medical or surgical cases, the veterinarian has little time to pursue a dental case properly. The veterinary dental technician is an essential team member and will find you the time. He or she extends your dental time by being able to clean, chart, and radiograph. Based on the technician's findings and your exam, you create the treatment plan, speak to your client, and perform the therapy.

- The veterinarian *must* arm teammates with the right equipment: a high-/low-speed delivery system (the power unit to energize high-/low-speed drills), a dental radiograph unit, an intraoral Polaroid, and home care supplies.

You Are the Pet's Advocate

- Our patients cannot speak for themselves, so they must live with oral pain. Pet owners do not want to live with a suffering animal. You *must* convince your client of the serious nature of dental disease, even though the animal may not be manifesting pain at that time. The pet ultimately benefits. When presenting exam findings to your client, speak as an ambassador for the animal. What type of treatment would the pet vote for?

- Veterinarians *must* increase their dental knowledge and skills through continuing education. You also *must* arm your staff by insisting on membership in the American Society of Veterinary Dental Technicians (ASVDT, 800-613-3647) and providing time to take the home study course and examination.

- Your technician *must* be able to evaluate each tooth on its own merit. If the technician's only job is to remove tartar off crowns, then dental disease will again prevail. The technician must be confident in his or her ability to bring abnormalities to the veterinarian's attention.

- An essential role of the technician is providing home care instruction. Performing teeth cleaning

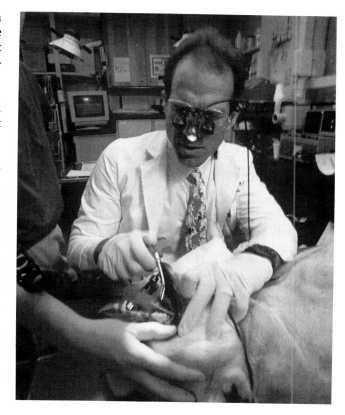

Fig. 1.3.

and sending the client home with a toothbrush is not practicing veterinary dentistry. Every teeth-cleaning visit *must* include an educational session with the pet's owner. Follow-up dental technician visits should be scheduled to make sure clients are brushing properly. Here, the technician saves the veterinarian time and becomes the most crucial team player as the home care educator.

Would you accept pain and infection in any other organ system without trying to diagnose and treat the problem? Why accept it in dentistry? Just because an overwhelming majority of veterinarians do not receive dental education, and do not have an understanding of dental disease, this does not mean we can turn our backs on what is necessary to good health.

A recent Minnesota study showed how dogs affected with periodontal disease had significant lesions in their kidneys and livers. *No other organ system is more important than the oral cavity. To ignore the oral cavity is to ignore your responsibility to your patient.*

Routine and consistent dental care will allow animals to do the following:

- Live longer—Periodontal disease may cause infections in the kidneys, liver, and heart, decreasing the pet's life span.

- Be more pleasant to live with—There is no reason for animals to have "doggie breath." Dogs with gingivitis or periodontitis have bad breath (halitosis) because bacteria attached where the teeth meet the gums. With proper treatment these bacteria will be removed and, with daily home care, disease prevented.

- Avoid dental discomfort—Dental disease will cause pain. Animals' dental nerve supplies are similar to those of humans. Because of their stoic nature, many animals will not manifest pain other than changes in behavior and general health.

  — Periodontal disease causes inflamed and painful gingiva.
  — Fractured teeth with pulpal exposure are painful initially and will lead to periapical inflammation.
  — Feline odontoclastic resorptive lesions, which affect 65 percent of all cats older than five years, may invade the dentin, resulting in extreme pain.

Dentistry Applies to All Age Groups

- Puppies and kittens—Young animals need care for retained deciduous teeth, orthodontic consultation, and correction of malocclusions that can cause pain. Home care must be emphasized at this age.

- Middle age—Periodontal disease, the most common small animal malady, starts when a pet is three years old unless the owner practices strict home care and agrees to periodic professional teeth cleaning.

- Old age—The challenge becomes saving and maintaining teeth that have lost support due to periodontal disease.

Understanding the Necessity of Dental Procedures

Getting your client to accept and understand the necessity for dental procedures is impossible if he or she perceives you are not convinced.

- Many veterinarians are guilty of presupposing what a client is willing to spend on a needed procedure. This inhibits them from making proper suggestions.

- Veterinarians who do not advocate the best in dental care would never tolerate the same amount of pathology in other parts of the body.

- If the best possible dentistry is not part of the overall service picture in your practice, then your patient is being neglected.

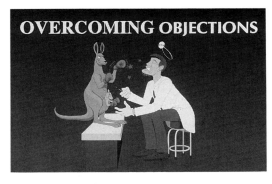

Fig. 1.4.

Veterinarian objections:

- "I do not have the time for that"—You *must* make the time. Do you have time for a heart condition but not a skin problem? Dental disease therapy is crucial to animals' well-being. Delegating nonveterinary responsibilities (taking and processing radiographs, charting, teeth cleaning, and giving home care instructions) to your trained staff frees up time for you to treat dental lesions that you have discovered.

- "My clients will not pay for that"—The dog or cat has the problem, not the client, and you need to focus on the patient's problem and pain, not the client's objections. Would the client pay for treatment of an ear infection or broken limb? You must convince your client that oral disease is as important as inflammation elsewhere.

- "My clients do not want this type of care"—This type of care is as basic to good health as any other care, and when presented properly, it will be accepted as quickly as other recommendations.

Client objections:

- Anesthesia—Clients worry about anesthesia. It is up to the veterinarian and staff to educate the client about the safety of anesthesia, to choose the safest anesthetic available, to qualify the patient through preanesthetic testing, and to monitor the pet once sedated.

- Cost—When educated on how important treatment is to the health of the pet, the client will usually not question the fees charged.

- Postoperative pain—Many dental procedures are painful. Nearly all periodontal surgery, root canal therapy, and oral surgery patients benefit from pain relief medication.

- Inability to provide home care—Your staff must teach clients methods of controlling periodontal disease.

Don't Stand in the Way of What Your Client Really Wants

As our profession has grown in sophistication, so have our clients. The many successful specialty groups functioning around the nation attest to our clients' willingness to use the newest techniques regardless of cost. Your clients come to you because you have established credibility with them. Tie this credibility to your newfound knowledge and belief in the need for the best dental care.

Ninety percent of your clients follow your recommendations. I have seen this happen in practice after practice with clients of every economic level. In my own practice, retirees living on social security and a modest pension agree to the most advanced procedures, as do those who are wealthy. Clients want—no, insist—on the best possible care for their pets.

Perseverance Pays

If your clients see how serious you are about their pets' oral problems, they will agree to your treatment plan. It may take several attempts to gain consent. Giving up after the first "no" gives the message that maybe dentistry is not really important.

- Imagine your client agreeing to what you recommend for dental care. Propose what you feel is necessary as if money never entered the decision, rather than basing your decision on your client's finances.

- An initial "I really can't afford this now" may actually have nothing to do with money. It may mean that the veterinarian or team member has not

given the client enough information about why the procedure must be done. You have a duty to your patient to help its owner overcome his or her concerns.

- For a client who drives a new car, an objection to needed dental work is not based on money. The problem is the client's perception of value. Some clients simply do not believe their pets' welfare is worth borrowing from the credit union or delaying vacations. We must educate clients about the importance of dental care.

- Need versus want—If your clients perceive that their animals *need* immediate dental care based on your presentation, they will agree and find a way to pay for it. If they feel you *want* to perform care not based on true need, they will object.

Ninety Percent of Communication Is Visual

The most effective communication uses visual aids. A pictorial display of pathology shows the lesions and helps you explain the need for therapy in a dramatic way. My most valuable tool for depicting a disease condition is a Polaroid close-up intraoral camera. This allows me to show my client immediately an enlarged picture of the pet's pathology.

THE MEMBERS OF THE DENTAL TEAM

A group of people is not a team. A team is a group of people geared toward the achievement of a goal. A relay team is a good example. The team members share a common goal, and they work together to achieve it. All members of an 800-meter relay team must do their part by running fast, passing the baton skillfully, and encouraging each other. While one person could run the distance, he or she could never compete with a team working together.

Everyone wants to be part of a winning team, especially one made up of dedicated, caring professionals with a common goal: fighting and overcoming disease so that companion animals can live longer, happier, painless lives. The enemy—dental disease—is a powerful opponent, one that is fed by a warm, moist, well nourished environment and encouraged by neglect, misinformation, and years of unchallenged growth to be as nasty as possible.

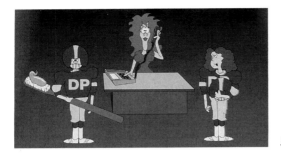

Fig. 1.5.

The Receptionist

Clients regard receptionists as part of the team protecting the health of their pets. Receptionists broadcast their interest in and knowledge of dentistry by their words and body language. Delivery of dental care usually starts (telephone appointment) and ends (collection of fees) with your receptionist. When the doctor or technician is not available for a dental examination, the receptionist needs to be able to "flip the lips" to show the client that there is gingivitis, periodontitis, or a fractured tooth in a pet that is being dropped off on the way to work.

The receptionist's personal positive feeling about dental home care is essential to your success. You can perform a wonderful periodontal surgical procedure and have the owner leave unhappy due to the receptionist's body language when collecting fees.

Your receptionist also handles the initial dental inquiry over the telephone. When asked how much a practice charges for "a dentistry," the answer must be "it depends on the degree of oral disease present." The receptionist should avoid quoting fees over the telephone. When the client receives the answer, "at Main Street Animal Hospital the fee for teeth cleaning is $125, which includes the teeth cleaning, anesthesia, antibiotics, and examination," then the client, patient, and animal hospital are getting shortchanged. In reality there is no such thing as "a dentistry": each dog or cat must have its teeth individually evaluated and treated, with fees specifically related to therapy performed.

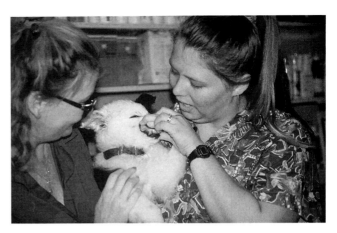

Fig. 1.6. Receptionist "flipping the lips" to examine dog's mouth in front of client.

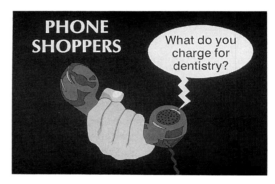

Fig. 1.8.

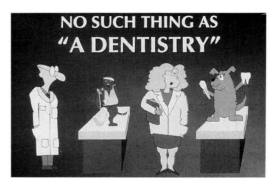

Fig. 1.9.

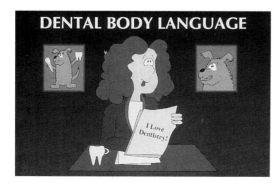

Fig. 1.7.

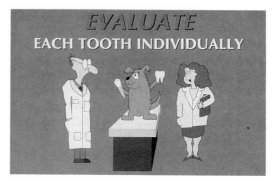

Fig. 1.10.

As you will see in Chapter 8, "Proposing Care," every dental case is different. The client that calls for a price quote does not know if his or her pet has grade one gingivitis or grade four periodontitis with mobile teeth. All the client knows is that the pet's breath smells bad. Giving one quote to handle all teeth-cleaning procedures may result in either necessary dental care being ignored or an upset owner finding out that 12 teeth with advanced periodontal disease were extracted without permission while the dog was anesthetized.

A better way of approaching the phone shopper, or an established client who is scheduling a teeth-cleaning appointment and wants to know what the fees will be, is to explain that the veterinarian must examine the pet's teeth one by one under anesthesia and evaluate dental radiographs before a treatment plan can be formulated and fees calculated.

To make sure your client is available when you are ready to discuss the treatment plan, schedule a *phone date* at a specific time. If the client can visit the practice instead calling, all the better. Showing clients dental pathology firsthand, while the animal is still anesthetized, is the best way of educating and securing appreciation for the diagnosis and proposed therapy. When the client cannot be there firsthand, Polaroid pictures are taken and used at the exit interview to explain the degree of pathology.

Let's imagine a six-year-old dog is left with your receptionist at 9 A.M. for dental care while the owner goes to work. The receptionist asks the owner to call at noon (on the dot) to find out what needs to be done after the you have "evaluated each tooth on its own merit." Before leaving the office, your receptionist or technician hands the owner a dental fee sheet with procedures to be done by noon circled. Items circled include the examination, preoperative blood testing (in the case of a six-year-old dog—CBC, BUN, ALT), anesthesia, pulse oximetry, and blood pressure monitoring, as well as grade two gingivitis teeth cleaning, polishing, antibiotic injection, and fluoride application.

Your staff must know that there is a telephone date set up at noon. Once you have performed a preanesthetic physical exam, they have the responsibility of performing a preoperative blood analysis, administering anesthesia under your direction, cleaning, charting, radiographing (if needed), and presenting pathology findings to you by 11:45. You again examine the mouth to confirm pathology and prepare a treatment plan to discuss with the owner. At noon your client calls and wants to know four things:

- What did you find?
- What can be done to treat it?
- What will it cost?
- When can the pet be picked up?

Receptionists have the responsibility of collecting dental fees. This can be a happy experience, with the client thanking all that helped, or a disaster, with your client feeling taken advantage of. The difference is how financial discussions are handled. Once you uncover pathology and gain approval from the client for treatment, someone must speak about fees. If your client has been properly educated, he or she wants therapy no matter what the cost. Discuss fees at this time; do not wait until the client picks up the pet *after* dental care. When the client agrees to a fee, the receptionist's job becomes easier—educate more and collect the agreed upon fee. Receptionists must be familiar with dental procedures. Clients will ask them why an apical repositioned flap had to be performed, and they expect a logical answer. Explain every item on the dental fee sheet to your receptionists. Also, make sure they understand the importance and use of home care products.

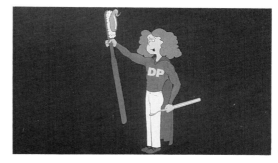

Fig. 1.11.

The Technician

Technicians are crucial players on the dental team. To create a successful dental practice, there has to be a technician whose main responsibility is dentistry. Practicing dentistry with an emphasis on home care, and frequent progress visits, creates enough dentistry in a small animal practice to justify a full-time dental technician. The technician's examination, communication, and therapy skills are vital for your dental team to win. How do you educate your technician? Start by asking the technician to join the American Society of Veterinary Dental Technicians. The society publishes an educational newsletter and produces a dental training video and examination.

A dental technician must know your procedures to better assist. Responsibilities include

- Promoting treatment plans and educating clients about procedures

- Charting the mouth/updating patient dental records on progress reports

- Performing teeth cleaning

- Helping the doctor with dental procedures

- Keeping the dental operatory clean and well stocked

- Keeping dental handpieces oiled and compressors maintained

- Taking oral radiographs

- Giving postoperative instructions

- Conducting periodic (weekly, monthly) home care progress visits

- Educating staff about oral hygiene products

Fig. 1.12. The American Society of Veterinary Dental Technicians provides education and training.

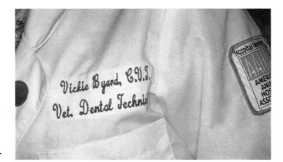

Fig. 1.13. A staff member should be trained to be the veterinary dental technician.

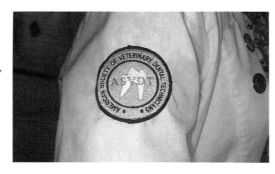

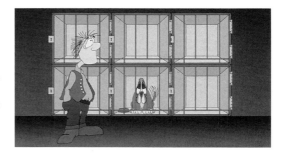

Fig. 1.14.

The Kennel Person

In most animal hospitals, pets are boarded when the owners go on vacation. What a wonderful opportunity to provide needed dental care. Insist that all boarders are examined *before* your client leaves. Show the pet owner the degree of oral pathology present and ask if it would be OK to clean the teeth while boarding. If more than grade one gingivitis is present, a telephone date will be necessary to approve advanced care.

Kennel staff are responsible for modeling the pet's home care through regular feeding and providing comfort, soothing words, and daily toothbrushing. If a boarder's owner does not bring a toothbrush to the hospital, the staff should encourage him or her to purchase one so the pet's teeth can be brushed daily. Again, the

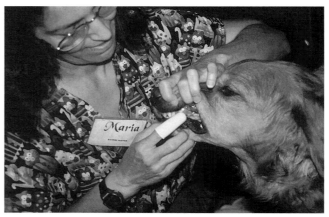

Fig. 1.15.

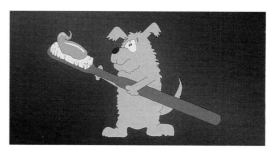

Fig. 1.16. Every patient should have its own toothbrush and toothpaste.

importance of oral care must be demonstrated to the owner. Daily toothbrushing must be included as part of your practice's hospitalization routine. When you go on a vacation or into the hospital, you brush your teeth daily, so why not the same care for small animals in your hospital?

The Veterinarian

The veterinarian is team captain and must believe that veterinary dentistry allows pets to live longer and healthier. The veterinarian must be comfortable recommending the best in dental care, including periodontal surgery, endodontics, and orthodontics to save teeth.

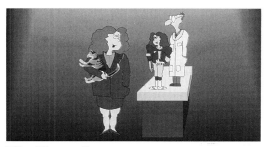

Fig. 1.17.

The Team Owner

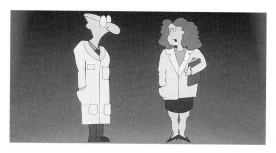

Fig. 1.18.

The pet's master is your team owner. Your clients pay for the services provided by the hospital staff and for the equipment used to diagnose and treat their pets. They spend 365 days each year with their animals. Owners make the choices: what to feed, whom to contact for veterinary care, what to buy for oral hygiene care, and how important dentistry will be to their pets' overall health. It is up to the veterinarian, receptionist, kennel person, and technician to convince the owner, who has not spent time in veterinary school, that proactive dental preventive care is a wise investment of time and money. Owners need to be trained to brush their pets' teeth daily and to agree to have frequent teeth cleanings or to accept compromised health. They also must be complimented for the important part they are playing in their pets' health.

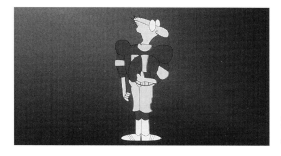

Fig. 1.20. Team Captain.

Veterinarian responsibilities include

- Setting proficiency goals and monitoring them
- Scheduling dental educational meetings
- Developing a highly trained and effective team to work with
- Providing patients the highest quality of dental care
- Setting fees
- Monitoring and controlling expenses

How to Hire the Best People for Your Dental Staff

- Be sure to hire "people persons" in all areas of the hospital. It is essential that team members are comfortable speaking to clients about dental matters.

- Offer competitive salaries and benefits. Learn what colleagues pay their staff and pay more. Ask employees what they want and give it to them.

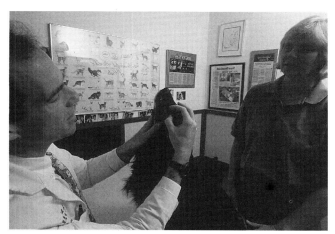

Fig. 1.19.

• Dental technicians need to be evaluated for competency. At our hospital the dental technician is not formally hired until he or she is able

— To chart a cat and dog mouth
— To perform teeth cleaning (all 12 steps) for grades one through four gum disease
— To take and process a complete set of oral films on a dog and cat within 20 minutes
— To send crowns to the laboratory
— To clean, lubricate, and oil the dental handpiece
— To drain compressors
— To make up dental surgical packs
— To give the client home care instructions stressing oral hygiene techniques for grades one and two teeth cleanings, grades three and four teeth cleanings, periodontal surgery, orthodontic care, and root canal therapy
— To understand indications for oral hygiene products based on grades of periodontal disease

READY, SET, FIRE—OR IS IT FIRE, SET, READY?

Creating a veterinary dental practice does not just happen. Unless you plan, it will never happen. Getting from the dream to reality is a journey well worth the travel. Steps along the way include

Desire

If with a snap of your fingers it were possible, what would you want your dental practice to look like? Without having to gain further education or make financial layouts, what level of dentistry would you perform? The same as you are doing now, or would you perform advanced endodontics, orthodontics, and periodontal guided tissue regeneration? Don't let that little voice in the back of your mind tell you advanced dental procedures would be too expensive for your clients to afford, or your clients would not want root canals for their pets. We will take care of client objections later in this book. What would *you* like to do? Make this your goal and formulate this as a mission statement for your dental practice.

How to Get from Where You Are Now to Where You Want to Be

If you try to "eat the elephant" all at once, you will become overwhelmed and discouraged. Split your dental dream into three attainable goals:

• The doable—Increase the quality of dentistry you are performing now: examine each tooth individually, chart all dental patients, take dental radiographs, act on pathology noted, and speak about dentistry to each client. Share your dental findings with the entire staff. Have them join the American Society of Veterinary Dental Technicians and take the home study dental course with them.

• Midrange goals—Do you want to perform root canal therapy or orthodontics? Once the doable is being practiced routinely, it's time to bite on bigger goals. Read whatever you can get your hands on about building the foundation of higher dental education. Team up with dentists with human practices. They are very willing to help.

• Dream goals—In dentistry there is always a new procedure or material to try. Perhaps you want to accept dental referrals from your colleagues. Maybe board certification is a dream goal. Dreams are reachable. Dental journals and continuing education seminars are full of ideas on how to move forward. Let your passion for dentistry drive the journey.

Dream Plan

Your dream in dentistry is attainable whatever the level. Getting from dream to reality takes desire, education, and equipment. Base the foundation of your plan on education. If you understand the why and how of a procedure, equipping your practice with the necessary supplies is easy. If you do not have the necessary education, then the best equipment is useless or, if used improperly, dangerous to your patient.

• Time horizon: understanding the principles of periodontics, endodontics, radiology, orthodontics, oral medicine, and surgery can take months to years. Do not let this scare you. When dentistry is cut up in small pieces, it becomes quite digestible.

• In your time horizon, set aside a month for learning about each of the above disciplines (nothing but periodontics for one month, endodontics the next, etc.). There are numerous sources of education, from books to veterinary dental magazines to computer on-line services to veterinary dental specialists who give hands-on wet labs. Annually, a major dental meeting features all disciplines of veterinary dentistry. Plan to "major" in one or two disciplines at each meeting. Write down concepts that you do not grasp so that you can ask for clarification from the dental specialists at the meetings or call them on the phone.

- Pick a mentor. Dentistry is too big a subject to learn completely by yourself. Ask a local dentist or veterinary dentist to be your helper. Most dentists with human practices love to help. Veterinary dentistry is something new for them: our patients routinely do not complain and are sleeping during procedures.

- Set up a budget for the financial support of your dream and journey. Keep track of what is spent and the increased income due to your enhanced dental practice. You will be amazed at how a little investment in equipment will produce practice profit.

Acting

- Approach every day as a way to accomplish your goals in your dental practice. Put your action plan into effect. There will be roadblocks along the way—hurdle over them! The payoff will be worth it.

- Examine each patient for lesions. Almost every dog and cat will have dental pathology. Practice how to present oral problems to your clients so that your proposed care can be performed and appreciated.

- *Fun is in the doing.*

HOW TO GET THE WORD OUT

Creating the veterinary dental practice is half of the battle. Informing others that you have a dental practice is the other. Heavy media blitzing, door-to-door soliciting, and lost leader come-ons ("veterinary dental care without anesthesia—$39") will not bring in quality clients who will provide necessary aftercare. For the most part, these clients take more time, complain more, and will leave your practice for the next veterinarian offering something for nothing.

Do not focus on pushing so many dental patients through the door that you treat only the superficial parts of the mouth. When you pay attention to *all* the oral pathology your current patients have, there is more than enough to keep your practice busy. You have a dental practice already. Each dog you examine actually has 42 patients in its mouth; cats have 30. Pay attention to the teeth of each patient no matter what that patient comes into the exam room for. When the pet is anesthetized, examine each tooth individually.

Internal Marketing

Everyone on your staff is responsible for getting the word out. Some hints include

- Tours through the office to explain the use of dental equipment

- An open house, where clients are invited to see an anesthetized dog or cat receiving dental care

- The entire staff wearing "pets need dental care too" buttons daily, not just for dental awareness month

- Dental models in each exam room

- Showing clients dental videos

- Sending out dental newsletters

- Asking clients if they want your staff to brush their pets' teeth while boarding

External Marketing

Press releases are tools to get the word out that you have created a dental practice. Writing a one- or two-page press release may seem like a simple assignment, yet a press release is a sophisticated, complex writing form that requires you to be both salesperson and storyteller.

Press releases that get published are those that best fill the needs, wants, and expectations of the local newspaper. Look for news in your practice. If you had no connection with your dental practice, what would be worth knowing about it?

The press release needs a peg. The peg is a unique angle from which you tell your story. The goal is to get the editor's interest. Rather than reporting on a fractured tooth you operated upon, title the press release "Root Canals in Dogs? You Bet!" Write a first sentence that sparks interest. Next, write about the most essential details, leaving the less important material at the bottom.

A second approach to external marketing is writing feature stories (Fig. 1.21). In a letter to the editor of the local newspaper, make suggestions for a good feature story about you and the practice. Supply interesting information about the type of dentistry you practice. The media are amazed that veterinarians perform periodontal surgery, orthodontic care, root canals, and restorative therapy.

Volunteer your dental services to the local zoo. When exotic animals are sedated for other procedures, have the zoo call you to evaluate and care for any oral

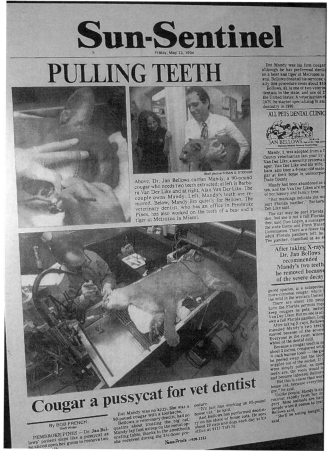

Fig. 1.21.

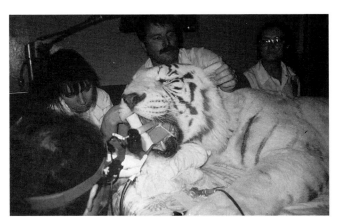

Fig. 1.22.

conditions. Call the press so it will cover the story when you are there.

Television is a third way to reach many people. There are numerous animal shows that will feature your newly created dental practice.

Keys to Veterinary Dental Practice Success

- Patient advocacy—The patient drives the team. Everyone's ultimate goal is to serve dog and cat patients. Insist that care be performed.

- Client-centered service—Work with your clients' ability to understand dental care and help them perform home care.

- Practice philosophy and values—Demand excellence in everything, including equipment, education, patient care, and follow-up.

- Continuous quality improvement—Practice this through evaluation and rewards.

2. ANATOMY AND NOMENCLATURE

*He that climbs a ladder must begin
at the first rung.*
—SIR WALTER SCOTT

NUMBER OF TEETH

Dogs

Dogs have 42 permanent teeth (Figs. 2.1–2.3).

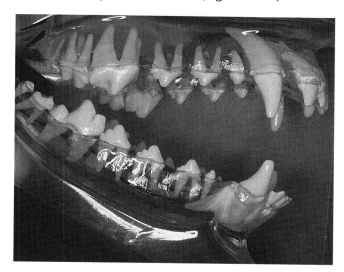

Fig. 2.1.

The **maxillary (upper) jaw** has

- Six incisors
- Two canines
- Eight premolars
- Four molars

The **mandibular (lower) jaw** has

- Six incisors
- Two canines
- Eight premolars
- Six molars

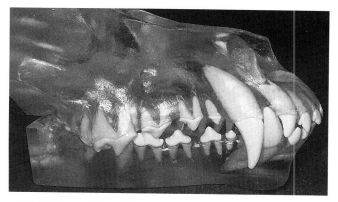

Fig. 2.2. *Dog maxilla and mandible.*

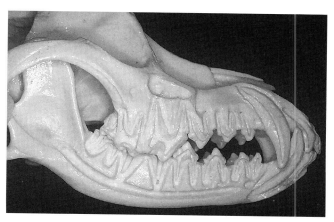

Fig. 2.3. *Dog maxilla and mandible with teeth cut away to reveal root canal system.*

Cats

There are 30 adult cat teeth in the normal mouth. The **maxillary jaw** (Figs. 2.4 and 2.5) has

- Six incisors
- Two canines
- Six premolars
- Two molars

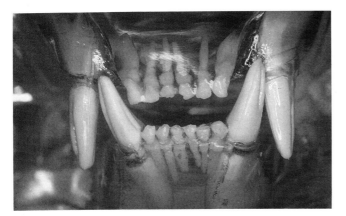

Fig. 2.4. Feline incisors and canines.

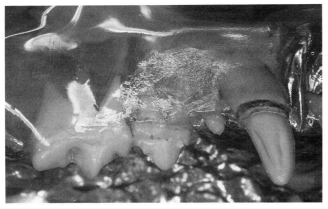

Fig. 2.5. Feline maxillary canine and premolars.

> ☼ **WHY IS THIS IMPORTANT?**
> When examining the mouth, if there are an abnormal number of teeth, investigate the reason. When teeth are missing, radiographs are needed to determine if they were present in the first place, if they are impacted, or if there is a fractured tooth root below the gum line that may cause future problems.

The **mandibular jaw** (Fig. 2.6) has

- Six incisors
- Two canines
- Four premolars
- Two molars

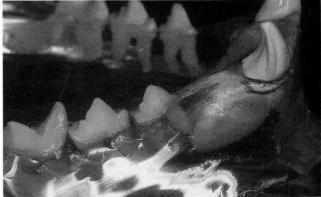

Fig. 2.6. Feline mandibular canines, premolars, and molars.

TYPES OF TEETH

There are four types of teeth in small animals: incisor, canine, premolar, and molar. Nature designed each to serve a special function.

Incisor teeth are the first teeth observed in the mouth (Figs. 2.7 and 2.8). In the normal dog and cat, there are six incisors in the maxilla and six in the mandible. Incisor teeth are used for grabbing food, tearing bits of tissue away from bone, and grooming. The occlusal surface on the incisor crown is called the incisal or cutting edge. Incisors are single-rooted teeth. Their size increases from central to lateral. Maxillary incisors are larger than mandibular.

Incisors are either identified by words (central, intermediate, lateral); numbers (first, second, third, or, depending on the quadrant, _01, _02, _03); or letters and numbers (I^2 = right maxillary second incisor).

There are two single-rooted **canine** teeth located in the maxilla and two in the mandible (Fig. 2.9). They are the longest teeth in the mouth. Only one-third of the canine tooth is exposed, with the remaining root firmly anchored in bone. The canines are curved backward and pointed to grasp and tear with great pressure.

Numbers can be used to identify canine teeth. In the Modified Triadan System, all canines end in a 4 (i.e., the maxillary right canine is tooth 104, maxillary left canine is tooth 204, mandibular left is tooth 304, mandibular right is 404).

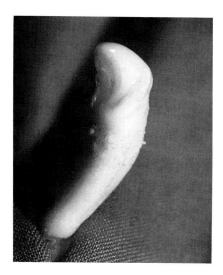

Fig. 2.7. Lateral view of extracted incisor showing crown and root.

Canines may also be identified with letters and numbers (^{1}C = left maxillary canine).

Premolar teeth have high central triangular elevations known as the principle cusps and smaller mesial and distal basal cusps (Fig. 2.10). Their sharp edges are used for shearing.

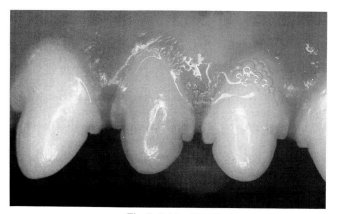

Fig. 2.8. Maxillary incisor crowns.

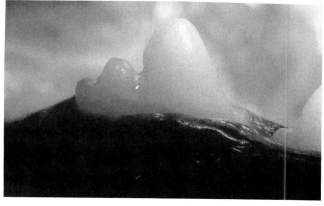

Fig. 2.10. Premolar tooth.

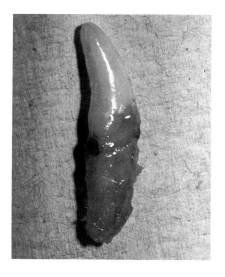

Fig. 2.9. Extracted canine tooth. Note crown and periodontal ligament–covered root.

Premolars have one, two, or three roots.

• First premolars in dogs and second maxillary premolars in cats are smaller single-rooted teeth.
• In the dog, the maxillary second and third premolars as well as the mandibular second, third, and fourth have two roots. In the cat, the maxillary third and mandibular second and third premolars are double rooted.

• The maxillary fourth is the largest premolar and has three roots. It is called a **carnassial tooth** because its function is to act with the mandibular first molar to cut food like a scissors.

• Using the Modified Triadan System, the first premolar can be numerically identified with a three-digit number ending with 5. Second through fourth premolars end in numbers 6 to 8. Premolars may also be identified by dental shorthand (^{2}P = left maxillary premolar).

In the dog, maxillary first and second **molars** have triple roots. Mandibular first, second, and third molars have double roots (Fig. 2.11). In the dog, molars have flat surfaces that are used for grinding; the first mandibular molar also has a cutting edge. The maxillary molar in the cat has a double root and is located distal to the maxillary fourth premolar.

Cats have only one maxillary and mandibular molar on each side of the mouth (Fig. 2.12).

In the Modified Triadan System, a three-digit number ending in 9 identifies the first molar; _10 and _11 signify the second and third molars.

HOW TO IDENTIFY TEETH

- Use *four words* to signify the type of tooth and where it is located in the mouth: i.e., "left maxillary fourth premolar" and "right mandibular lateral incisor."

- Use *three numbers* to identify teeth (Fig. 2.13). In the **Modified Triadan System**, tooth 208 is the left maxillary fourth premolar.

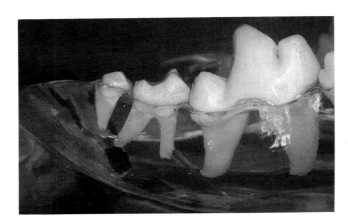

Fig. 2.11. Canine mandibular molar teeth.

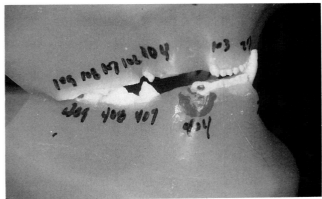

Fig. 2.13. Feline dental model with tooth numbers. Courtesy of Pharmacia & Upjohn Animal Health.

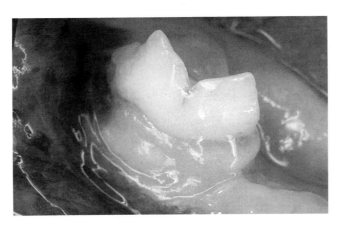

Fig. 2.12. Feline mandibular molar tooth.

— The *first digit* of the three-digit number signifies quadrant location and whether a tooth is primary or secondary.
— The 100 series is used for right maxillary teeth, 200 for left maxillary, 300 for left mandibular, and 400 for right mandibular dentition.
— Five hundred, 600, 700, and 800 series are used for primary teeth.
— Second and third digits signify a specific tooth. Central incisors end in 1. Moving distally, the next tooth ends in 2, followed by 3. Canines end in 4. First premolars end in 5. First molars end in 9.

- Dental "shorthand" (*letters and numbers*)

— Letters: *I* = incisor, *C* = canine, *P* = premolar, *M* = molar.
— Numbers 1–4 indicate first, second, third, or fourth.

Where the number is placed around the letter indicates which quadrant. Example: P³ would indicate right maxillary third premolar.

STRUCTURE

Each normal tooth consists of a crown and one or more roots. The size, location, and shape of the crown and the size and number of roots determine a tooth's function (Figs. 2.14 and 2.15).

Teeth are composed of a portion above the gum line called the **crown**, and a section below the gum line called the **root**. The end of each root is called the **apex**. A small opening can be found in the apex called the **apical foramen**, which allows passage of blood vessels and nerves into the tooth. The crown and root meet at the **cervix** or **neck** of the tooth.

Enamel, the hardest mineralized tissue found in the body, covers the crown, bulges at the base (the enamel bulge), and ends at the **cemento-enamel junction (CEJ)**, located at the neck of the tooth where the crown ends and **cementum** covering the normal root begins.

Enamel is produced when the dog or cat is young and is completed by four months of age. Enamel is a crystalline structure of hydroxyapatite that hardens with age. When enamel is damaged, the body will not repair it by making more, although surface mineralization can occur.

Pulp is composed of connective tissue, nerves, blood, and lymphatic vessels. It is responsible for the tooth's early life support. The pulp has four main functions. It

- Forms dentin
- Gives nutrition to the dentin through tubules
- Supplies nerve sensitivity to the dentin
- Protects itself through the secretion of reparative dentin in response to injury

The **pulp cavity** located in the crown is called the **pulpal chamber**, and in the root, the **root canal**. Each root has one root canal. Multirooted teeth have two or three root canals, which communicate with each other. Nourishment enters the pulp through the apical foramina located at the root tip. In the young dog or cat, the apex is open. At about one and a half years of age, the apex closes, and an apical delta forms at the root tip. The apical delta contains small canals where pulpal tissue enters the tooth.

In the young dog or cat, root canal contents called **pulp** occupy most of the tooth. Pulp produces **dentin**. As the animal matures, more dentin is laid down, causing pulp to be compressed. Greater than 80 percent of the mature tooth is composed of **dentin**. Dentin is softer than enamel and is porous. **Primary dentin** is produced by pulp tissue located in the tooth's center. Once a tooth erupts, **secondary dentin** continues to be

produced. As more dentin is created, the wall thickens, and pulp size shrinks.

Within the dentin, small tubules communicate from the pulp toward the enamel. These tubules transmit sensations of pain, temperature, and pressure. Bacteria from exposed crown or root surfaces can travel down these tubules, reach the pulp, and cause infection or pulpitis.

When the crown is mildly traumatized, or when sections of enamel are worn, **reparative, tertiary,** or **sclerotic dentin** may be produced to protect the pulp.

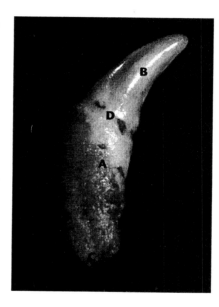

Fig. 2.14. Outside of canine tooth: A = root, B = crown, C = root apex, and D = cemento-enamel junction.

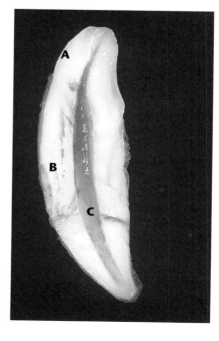

Fig. 2.15. Cutaway section of tooth: A = enamel, B = dentin, and C = pulp.

Reparative dentin is produced at an accelerated rate. Often stained darker than primary dentin, it appears as shiny black or brown areas over the surface of worn teeth.

> ☧ **WHY IS THIS IMPORTANT?**
>
> Enamel fractures that expose dentin and do not directly reveal the pulp may still cause infection and discomfort to the animal through transmission of sensation and bacteria to the pulp.

ERUPTION TIMES	INCISORS	CANINES	PREMOLARS	
Molars				
Primary teeth (weeks)				
Dog	2-4	3-5	4-12	
Cat	2-4	3-4		
Adult teeth (months)				
Dog	3-5	4-7	4-6	4-7
Cat	3-5	4-5	4-6	4-5

DENTAL ERUPTION

Dogs and cats are similar to humans in that they are born without visible teeth. The first teeth to be noticed in a puppy or kitten are referred to as **primary, temporary, baby, milk,** or **deciduous** teeth. Primary teeth are normally shed to make way for **adult,** or **secondary,** teeth. Shedding or exfoliation of the primary teeth takes place between three and eight months of age in most breeds.

Dogs have 28 deciduous teeth. Adult incisors erupt at three to five months. Adult canines show between four and seven months. First premolars emerge as secondary teeth at 100–150 days. The second and third premolars appear around 150 days, followed by the fourth premolars at 135–185 days and the secondary molars between 140 and 220 days.

> ☧ **WHY IS THIS IMPORTANT?**
>
> Knowing when teeth are supposed to be present is helpful in determining the age of a puppy or kitten. If the deciduous teeth are present without adult teeth showing, the puppy or kitten is probably younger than six months.

Cats' deciduous teeth begin to show at 11–15 days, and all should be present by eight weeks. There are 26 deciduous cat teeth. The adult incisors emerge between three and five months, soon followed by canines (four to five months), premolars (four to six months), and molars (four to five months).

QUADRANTS

An imaginary midline divides the arch of each jaw into mirror halves. The two arches, split into halves, create four sections called **quadrants.** The four quadrants are identified as maxillary right, maxillary left, mandibular right, and mandibular left.

TOOTH SURFACES

Each tooth has multiple surfaces.

Labial—Surface of anterior teeth positioned adjacent to the lip

Lingual (mandibular tooth) or **palatal** (maxillary tooth)—That surface that faces toward the tongue or palate

Distal—Surface or side of a tooth that faces away from the dental arch's midline

Mesial—Surface that is closest to or faces the dental arch's midline

Buccal—Surface of posterior teeth adjacent to the cheek or lip. **Vestibular** is sometimes used as a synonym for buccal.

Facial—Both the buccal and labial surfaces

Occlusal—Chewing surface of a posterior tooth

Coronal—In direction of the crown tip

Contact or proximal—Surface facing adjoining teeth in the same arch

Interproximal space—Space between two facing proximal surfaces

Apical—Directed toward the apex, or tip of the root

Maxillary—Relating to the upper jaw

Mandibular—Relating to the lower jaw

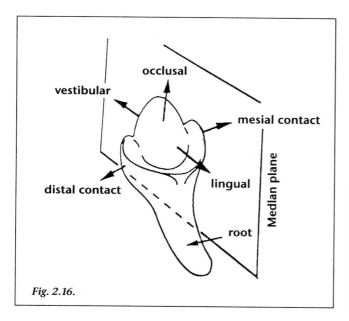

Fig. 2.16.

The **periodontal ligament's** fibroelastic network suspends the tooth in alveolar bone. Respective ends of this ligament are buried in cementum and alveolar bone. Radiographically, the normal periodontal ligament appears as a black line surrounding the root.

The **alveolar process** is bone that forms and supports tooth sockets. The process consists of supporting alveolar bone and an inner socket wall composed of thin, compact bone called the cribiform plate.

> ꙮ**WHY IS THIS IMPORTANT?**
>
> Periodontal disease is the most common small animal problem. Understanding the anatomy of the periodontium will help with the diagnosis of pathology that may lead to impaired patient health, discomfort, and tooth loss.

PERIODONTAL TISSUES

Periodontal tissues are composed of gingiva, cementum, periodontal ligament, and alveolar bone (Fig. 2.17). **Gingiva** covers the bones that surround teeth.

- **Attached gingiva** is tightly bound to the periosteum of the alveolar bone. Healthy attached gingiva is required for maintenance of periodontal health. Coronal to the attached gingiva at the cemento-enamel junction is the **marginal** or **free gingiva**, which normally touches enamel.

- The **gingival sulcus** is a space between a tooth and free gingiva.

- The **mucogingival line (MGL)** separates attached gingiva from loose alveolar mucosa.

- **Subgingival** refers to the area below the gum line toward the apex.

- **Supragingival** refers to the area above the gum line on the crown.

Cementum covers the roots and is where the periodontal ligament attaches to the tooth. Unlike enamel, cementum deposition occurs throughout life.

The **cemento-enamel junction (CEJ)** is located where the crown terminates on the root surface. It is also the location where healthy gingiva attaches to the tooth.

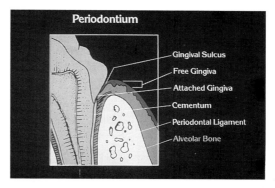

Fig. 2.17.

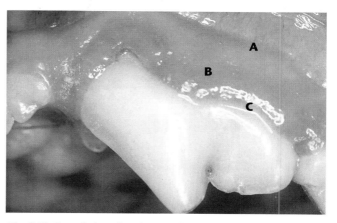

Fig. 2.18. Buccal view of canine maxillary fourth premolar. A = mucogingival line (MGL), B = attached gingiva, C = free gingival margin.

Deep depressions in the jawbones are called **alveolar sockets** (Fig. 2.19), which contain tooth roots. The cribiform plate covers the alveolar socket and appears as a dense white line on radiographs. Often, when teeth are lost due to periodontal disease, bone will fill in, eliminating the socket.

HOW THE MOUTH PROTECTS ITSELF

The teeth of dogs and cats are designed to be self-cleaning. The tongue, lips, and cheeks help to mechanically remove bacteria from the oral cavity. Friction created from eating hard food also assists in keeping teeth clean. In the healthy mouth, intact gingival tissues around the teeth provide protection against bacteria colonizing and taking control of the oral cavity. Unfortunately, if oral hygiene is not practiced, plaque accumulates at and below the free gingival margin, causing inflammation.

Saliva contains a hydrogen peroxide–based antibacterial system. Saliva helps to protect the mouth by washing bacteria away. It enters the oral cavity through duct openings located under the tongue and lateral to the maxillary fourth premolar and maxillary second premolar. In addition to lubricating food, saliva contains substances (lysozymes) that interfere with bacterial growth and adherence to the tooth.

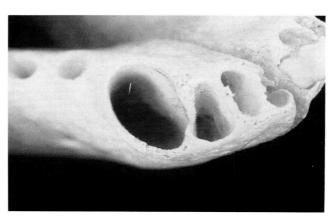

Fig. 2.19. Mandibular incisor, canine, and premolar alveolar sockets.

Carnivore saliva has a pH of about 7.5, which encourages the deposition of bacteria-laden plaque. *The heaviest plaque accumulation occurs close to the areas that salivary glands exit.* Although any tooth surface will support plaque and calculus, *most plaque occurs on the buccal (cheek) surfaces of the maxillary fourth premolar,* followed by the labial surface of the canines. The least affected areas are on the lingual (tongue side) surfaces of the mandibular teeth.

3. ORAL EXAMINATION

Never take anything for granted.
—BENJAMIN DISRAELI

WHY, WHEN, AND HOW TO EXAMINE DOG AND CAT MOUTHS

An examination is a process of observing both normal and abnormal conditions. Whose job is it when it concerns dentistry? It's *everyone's*. The receptionist, technician, kennel person, veterinarian, and pet owner have joint responsibility each time an animal is handled to examine the mouth. Why? Because our animals cannot speak for themselves. Without our help they suffer quietly with the pain of periodontal inflammation, fractured teeth, or feline odontoclastic resorption. Meticulous attention to detail is the basis of diagnosing dental disease.

Dentistry differs from other areas of medicine, such as orthopedics, ophthalmology, or dermatology, where patients present with obvious signs of problems. Other than halitosis, which many clients accept as normal, our patients do not show evidence of dental disease until it is advanced. Most small animals with fractured teeth, oral cancer, grades three and four periodontal disease, and malocclusions continue to eat and drink without difficulty. This makes the oral examination and creation of a therapy plan essential to delivering companion animal dental care. Remember, a majority of client-owned dogs and cats are walking around with significant oral disease requiring immediate attention. Without an oral examination, nothing meaningful can be accomplished.

Step 1: Where Does the Examination Start? With Listening

The dental history is divided into two parts:

- A review of past dental history

- A review of current problems

Past dental history reveals information about your patient's dental problems and treatment. Frequency of the pet's dental care and the owner's perceptions of that care may be indicators of his or her future behavior. The client's eagerness and ability to perform home care must be discussed.

The review of the dental history ultimately focuses on your patient's present problem, with the chief complaint recorded on the dental chart. Encourage your client to discuss all aspects of the current problem. Questions to ask:

- When did you first notice the problem?

- What signs of the problem, if any, does your animal show?

- What does your pet normally eat? Generally, companion animals that are fed soft food or their owners' diets are more prone to periodontal disease than those on hard food.

- What are your animal's favorite chew toys? Some dogs and cats chew on their cages, chains, cow hooves, abrasive tennis balls, or stones when bored. Investigation of the cause of an injury is important because what patients chew on may continue to cause lesions once your treatment is concluded unless your client is educated about potential harm.

- Are there problems with drinking or swallowing?

- Is there any rubbing of the face with paws or on carpeting? This may indicate pain or inflammation.

- Is there any dropping of food?

• Is there drooling?

• Does your pet grind its teeth? This happens especially in cats.

Step 2: General Health Exam

Before you center attention on the mouth, perform a general examination of the rest of the animal's body. This includes a checkup of the eyes, ears, skin, heart, lungs, and abdomen. Depending on the animal's age and condition, if anesthesia is planned, blood, urine, stool, and intestinal parasite tests; an electrocardiogram; and chest radiographs are performed.

Step 3: Head Exam—without Anesthesia

The breath of a dog or cat normally has a pleasant, slightly sweet odor. *Halitosis* and *fetor oris* are terms used to indicate offensive breath. Common reasons for halitosis include poor oral hygiene resulting in periodontal disease, orthodontic malocclusions resulting in perforations of the gingiva, oral abscesses from fractured teeth, dying tissue due to oral cancer, systemic disease, and nasal and respiratory infection.

Compare sides of the head. Does one side appear different than the other? Look at the eyes. If one appears to be bulging, this may be due to glaucoma or a tumor behind the eye. If skin below the eye is inflamed, look for a fractured maxillary third or fourth premolar tooth (Fig. 3.1).

Lymph nodes can become enlarged secondary to infection or neoplasia. **Sublingual** nodes are located in the sublingual triangle between the chin, hyoid bone, and digastric muscle. These nodes drain the skin of the chin, tip of the tongue, mandibular incisors, and lower lip.

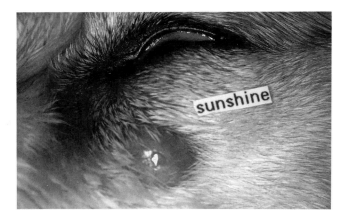

Fig. 3.1. Swelling under the eye, which usually indicates an abscess of the maxillary fourth premolar.

The **submandibular nodes** are located between the two digastric muscles and the lower border of the mandible in the submandibular triangle. The submandibular nodes drain the upper and lower lips, the palate, the body of the tongue, and all teeth except mandibular incisors, then drain into the cervical lymph nodes.

Generalized inflammation produces enlarged lymph nodes that are tender, firm, and freely mobile. Nodes that are stone hard, nontender, and nonmobile may be indicative of neoplasia.

Examine the skin overlying the maxilla and mandible. Check for swelling, tenderness, masses, and discharge.

The **initial intraoral exam** can be performed next if your patient allows. When the dog or cat resists with aggression, do not attempt to examine further. Most small animals will allow a gentle examination of the mouth. *Gentle* should be the operative term. Pets remember pain and will not allow future examinations if they are hurt.

CHECKING THE TEETH

First, evaluate the bite, or the relationship of the maxilla to the mandible.

• Does the dog or cat have an overbite, underbite, open bite, or normal bite?

• How do the incisor teeth line up? Is there a level or wry bite?

• Gently retract the sides of the lips backward, exposing cheek teeth. How do these teeth interdigitate?

Next, try to visually evaluate each tooth.

• Are there tooth fractures?
• Are there areas of periodontal inflammation?
• Are there missing, extra, or mobile teeth?
• Show your clients their pets' maxillary cheek teeth. Most clients only see the incisors, which do not accumulate calculus readily. A majority of dogs and cats older than two years have calculus touching the maxillary fourth premolar gingiva, which causes inflammation and necessitates immediate care.

The **temporomandibular joint** is examined by placing a finger directly below the external ear canal and manually moving the jaw up and down. Pain experienced during palpation is indicative of disease. Conditions common to the temporomandibular joint include arthritis, ankylosis, luxation, and fracture.

Place a stethoscope over the temporomandibular joint to hear abnormal popping, clicking, and grating sounds.

CHECKING FOR MOBILITY

Normally, teeth are not mobile. Mobility denotes defects in alveolar support. Mobility testing is performed by placing pressure on the coronal surfaces of the teeth with a scaler or curette.

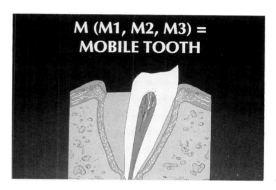

Fig. 3.2.

Mobility of teeth may be classified as follows:

- **M1** indicates slight mobility. The tooth can be moved 1 mm in a horizontal direction.
- **M2** indicates moderate mobility. The tooth can be moved 2 mm in a horizontal direction.
- **M3** indicates marked mobility. The tooth can be depressed vertically into its socket as well as horizontally.

Step 4: Examination of the Mouth—under General Anesthesia

The tongue, buccal mucosa, palate, and oropharynx are checked for areas of inflammation and abnormal growths. The periodontal examination includes visual and probe inspection of the gingiva and radiography of the supporting bone.

CHECKING THE GINGIVA

Healthy gingiva is firm, coral pink, and knife edged. Unhealthy gingiva is red, soft, and swollen. Gingiva has three anatomic divisions: free, attached, and alveolar mucosa.

- **Free gingiva** is the unattached coronal portion surrounding the tooth. Its outer surface normally

appears knife edged. The inner surface forms a 1- to 3-mm sulcus between the free gingival margin and attached gingiva.

- **Attached gingiva** lies apical to the free gingiva and normally forms a nonmovable tight cuff around the tooth.

- Movable **alveolar mucosa** lies apical to the attached gingiva. The **mucogingival line** demarcates attached gingiva from alveolar mucosa.

The periodontium is examined through a series of methods. First, the depth of the gingival sulcus around each tooth is determined by systematic probing. A sulcular depth greater than 2 mm in the dog and 1 mm in the cat is abnormal and recorded in the patient's chart.

Pocketing, which is an abnormal sulcular depth, indicates the presence of periodontal disease (Figs. 3.3 and 3.4).

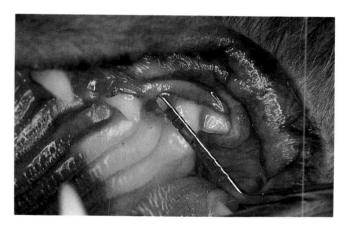

Fig. 3.3. Periodontal probe prior to insertion.

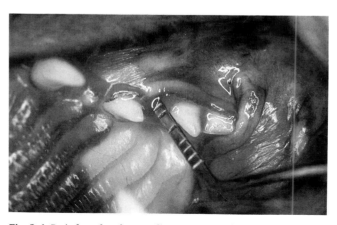

Fig. 3.4. Periodontal probe revealing a 4-mm pocket.

Appearance of **normal gingiva:**

- Coral pink with stippling of the attached gingiva
- Between the incisor teeth, pointed papillae filling the interproximal spaces
- Margins sloping coronally to a thin edge
- Firm to palpation, with the attached portion connected to alveolar bone
- Sulcus depths less than 2 mm in the dog and 1 mm in the cat

Appearance of **abnormal gingiva:**

- Any purulent or bloody discharge
- Recession of the gingival margin apical to the cemento-enamel junction
- Supragingival or subgingival calculus and plaque

  — Calculus is calcified dental plaque that adheres to the crown and/or root surface.
  — Supragingival calculus is often found in abundance on the maxillary fourth premolars and canines, adjacent to the salivary gland ducts.
  — Subgingival plaque can be found anywhere in the dentition and is the main instigator of periodontal disease.

Recognition of dental plaque and its pathologic potential on the gingival tissue is of utmost importance to dental health.

CHECKING FOR FURCATION INVASIONS
In multirooted teeth, bone loss may progress to bifurcation or trifurcation if the roots are involved. Involvement is classified as

- **Class 1—incipient bone loss,** where the periodontal probe enters 1 mm into the furcation
- **Class 2—definite bone loss,** where the periodontal probe enters 3–5 mm into the furcation
- **Class 3—through and through bone loss,** which extends through the furcation

PERIODONTAL PROBING
The periodontal probe is the most useful tool for evaluating the periodontal status of a patient. It must be used in all dental examinations. Most pockets are not reliably detected or measured by visual or radiographic examination. Periodontal pockets are soft tissue changes. Radiographs indicate areas of bone loss where pockets may occur but do not show pockets or indicate pocket depth. The only accurate method of detecting and evaluating periodontal pockets is careful exploration with a periodontal probe.

A sulcus depth greater than 2 mm in the dog and 1 mm in the cat is considered pathologic and called a **pocket.** Probing gives a "dipstick" numerical evaluation of the depth of the gingival sulcus or pocket. A record of pocket depth is kept in the patient's chart. Two methods of probing are circumferential and spot probing:

- **Circumferential probing** means that the probe is used in at least four places (two buccal, two lingual) around the sulcus or pocket. This method eliminates inaccurate depth readings when subgingival calculus is present or if areas of vertical bone loss exist.

- **Spot probing** is the insertion and withdrawal of the probe at single areas. Single areas do not represent the entire tooth. Inaccurate readings may be obtained when subgingival calculus is present and when there are varying bone loss depths around a tooth.

PROBING DEPTH AND ATTACHMENT LOSS
The **clinical** or **probing depth** is the distance that a periodontal probe penetrates into the sulcus or pocket. It is the depth between the base of the pocket and the gingival margin. This depth will depend on factors such as the size of the probe, the force introduced, and the direction of penetration.

Determining the attachment level (or attachment loss) is a better evaluation of periodontal disease because it takes gingival recession into account. The level of attachment is determined by measuring the distance from the cemento-enamel junction (CEJ) to the bottom of the pocket. When the gingival margin coincides with the cemento-enamel junction, the level of attachment and the pocket depth are equal. When the gingival margin is located apical to the cemento-enamel junction, the loss of attachment will be greater than the pocket depth.

Following are some examples of the clinical significance of probing depth and attachment loss:

- A Labrador retriever whose maxillary canine has a 9-mm pocket depth and an 8-mm attachment loss from grade four periodontal disease may require an apical reposition flap to decrease the pocket depth and save the tooth (number 1 in Fig. 3.5).

- A boxer with a 7-mm pocket depth and a 5-mm attachment gain (distance from the CEJ to the gingival margin) secondary to gingival hyperplasia should undergo a gingivectomy to eliminate the pseudopocket (number 2 in Fig. 3.5).

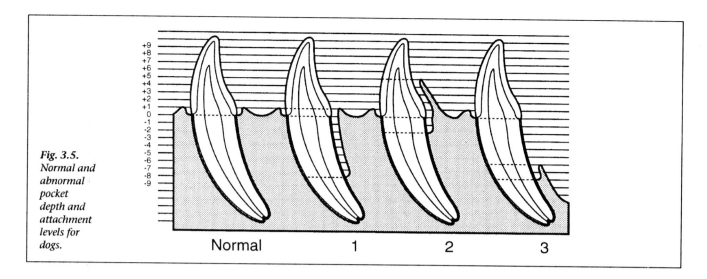

Fig. 3.5.
Normal and
abnormal
pocket
depth and
attachment
levels for
dogs.

Normal   1   2   3

- A poodle with a 2-mm pocket depth and an 8-mm attachment loss around the maxillary canine due to gingival recession has a normal probing depth but significant attachment loss. Extraction may be the treatment of choice (number 3 in Fig. 3.5).

THE IMPORTANCE OF INDIVIDUAL TOOTH INSPECTION

The hallmark of a thorough dental examination is individual tooth inspection. In essence the normal dog has 42 patients in its mouth, and the normal cat, 30. Global exams based on a cursory evaluation of the mouth will result in poor dental care due to unintentional neglect of pathology. The dental exam must be done systematically—each tooth must be fully evalu-

ated, including the gingival support, and findings recorded on a dental chart. Adequate lighting, magnification, and a sharp number five explorer are necessary exam tools.

Whenever an abnormality is found, seek the cause and formulate a treatment plan if the lesion has potential to cause harm. The veterinarian is the pivotal player here. Imagine you are presented with the oral problem depicted in Figures 3.6 and 3.7. Your technician notes an area of inflammation apical to the left maxillary third incisor during a teeth-cleaning examination. You have two choices as a veterinarian: to leave the lesion alone or to pursue treatment.

If you leave it alone, your patient's lesion may cause infection and discomfort when the animal eats with a mobile tooth. Hopefully, you will choose to pursue further diagnostics. The next step is to radiograph the

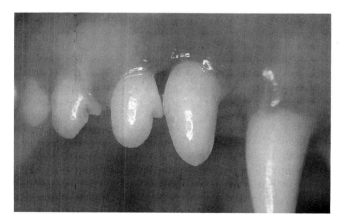

Fig. 3.6. Inflammation apical to left maxillary third incisor.

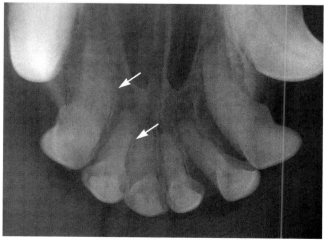

Fig. 3.7. Radiograph revealing marked bone loss around the left maxillary intermediate and lateral incisors (arrows).

tooth. The area of bone loss noted should lead you either to extract the tooth or to perform advanced periodontal care. Fortunately, when we encountered this problem, we were able to save the tooth through splinting and guided tissue regeneration.

THE DENTAL CHART

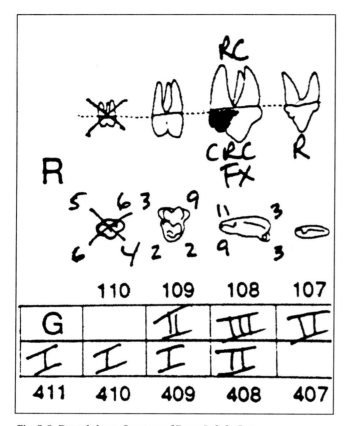

Fig. 3.8. Dental chart. Courtesy of DentaLabels Company.

Why Chart?

Abnormal clinical and radiographic findings are noted on the dental chart as a permanent part of the patient's record. Recording the condition of all teeth, as well as soft and hard tissues, is necessary for a number of reasons:

- It promotes quality care. Charting of existing conditions provides basic information for an accurate, comprehensive treatment plan.

- It facilitates communication with other veterinarians.

- It represents legal documentation of care delivered or declined.

The dental chart is a permanent record of the what, why, when, and what is next in a patient's dental care. It should include

- Dental history
- Skull type (brachycephalic—flat faced, mesocephalic—medium faced, dolichocephalic—long nosed)
- Oral hygiene—is there plaque and calculus present?
- Tooth abnormalities
- Radiographic findings
- Results of periodontal examination for inflammation, gingival edema, sulcular probe depths, recession, hyperplasia, and mobility
- Proposed treatment
- Actual treatment
- Future treatment plans
- Home care instructions including proposed recheck appointments

FOUR-HANDED CHARTING

Anesthesia is essential for complete examination and charting. To evaluate each tooth individually on its own merit, complete immobilization is necessary.

Four-handed charting is the fastest and most efficient way to chart. One person examines the mouth, and the other records information on the chart. The examiner begins by saying, "100 series," and then says, "101," which is the maxillary right central incisor. After noting any abnormalities, the examiner then moves distally until the right maxillary quadrant is completed. The right mandibular quadrant (400 series) follows, and then the animal's head is rotated for the 200 and 300 series. Each tooth must be charted completely, including periodontal probe depths, before the next tooth is examined.

Charting Steps

1. Charting begins with general evaluation of the gingiva for presence of calculus on the buccal and labial areas of the teeth. Grading is 1 = slight, 2 = moderate, 3 = heavy calculus.
2. Next, examine the mouth for missing teeth. Missing teeth are circled on the chart.
3. Enamel, dentin plus enamel, and pulpal fractures are observed and noted.
4. A periodontal probe with millimeter gradations is inserted at the interface between the free gingiva and tooth surface. The probe is gently pressed down to the bottom of the sulcus, then "walked" around the tooth, and measurements are noted at the four corners of each tooth. Also noted are

attachment loss depths from the cemento-enamel junction to the pocket base.

5. Other lesions are observed and noted.

A dental chart must be user friendly. When choosing one for your dental practice, look for ease of noting general oral problems (halitosis, rubbing of the face, drooling, bleeding, problems with opening or closing the mouth) as well as oral pathology, including ailments above and below the gum line.

There are several dental charts commercially available (Figs. 3.9–3.11).

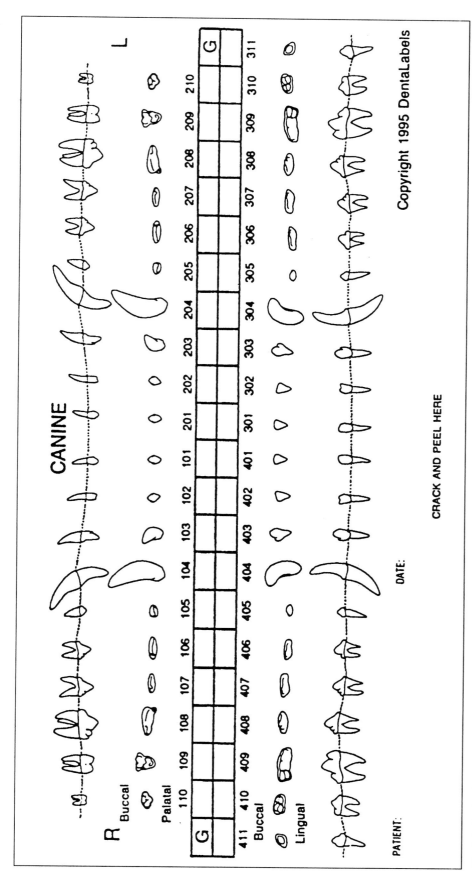

Fig. 3.9. Canine dental chart. Courtesy of DentaLabels Company.

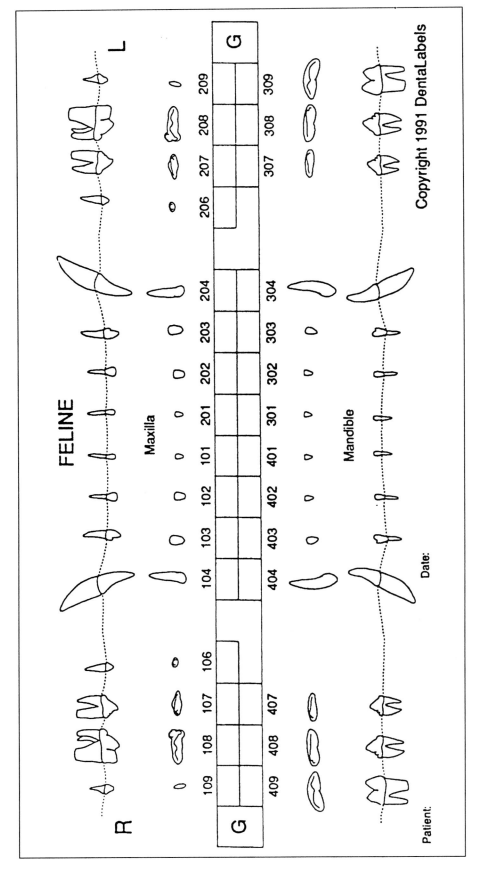

Fig. 3.10. *Feline dental chart. Courtesy of DentaLabels Company.*

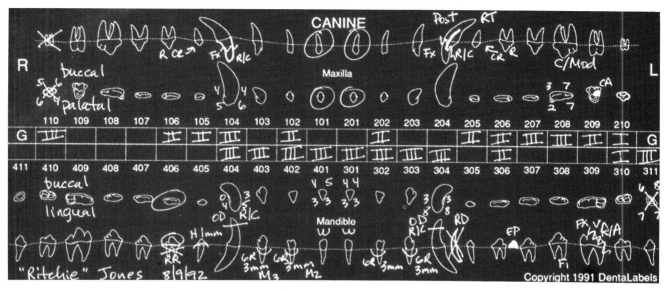

Fig. 3.11. Completed canine dental chart. Courtesy of DentaLabels Company.

Charting Shorthand

On dental charts, letters are placed over the diagram of a tooth to indicate the type of pathology noted. Some examples:

AB—abrasion. A pathologic wearing away of the dental tooth surface by friction of a foreign material (Figs. 3.12 and 3.13). Examples: tennis balls (dirt gets trapped in the fiber, the dog chews or spins the ball in its mouth, and this wears down the tooth surface), hair coat, and metal furniture.

A—adontia. Absence of a tooth or multiple teeth. Also called hypodontia or oligodontia (Fig. 3.14).

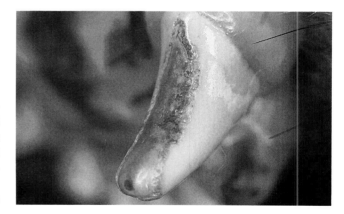

Fig. 3.13. Worn area on distal surface of canine tooth caused by wear from fence chewing.

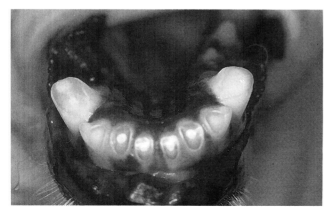

Fig. 3.12. Abraded incisor area secondary to biting on hair coat.

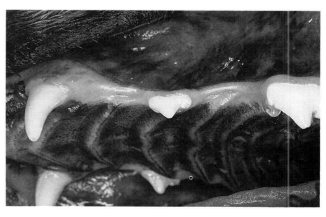

Fig. 3.14. Dog missing maxillary first and third premolars.

AK—ankylosis. Fusion of cementum with alveolar bone (Fig. 3.15).

ACB—anterior crossbite. Malocclusion where one or more of the maxillary incisors lie distal to mandibular incisors (Fig. 3.16). Anterior crossbite only affects the incisor teeth.

ARF—apical repositioned flap. Surgical procedure used to replace gingiva apically to eliminate periodontal pocket(s).

AT—attrition. A pathological wearing away of the tooth caused by an opposing tooth (Fig. 3.17).

AV—avulsion. The separation of a tooth from its alveolus.

BNC—base narrow canine. Mandibular canine penetrating maxilla (Fig. 3.18).

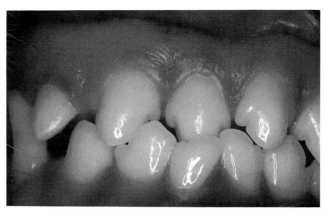

Fig. 3.16. Anterior crossbite. Central maxillary incisor positioned distal to mandibular central incisor.

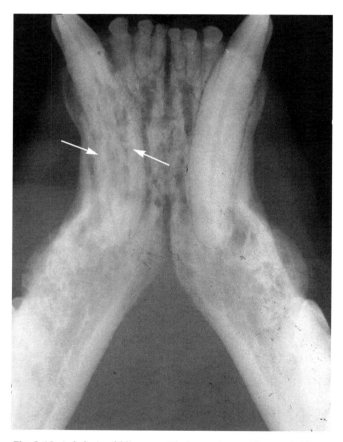

Fig. 3.15. Ankylosis of feline mandibular canine root (arrows). *Note absence of periodontal ligament space.*

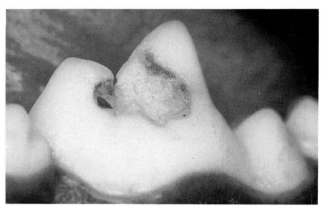

Fig. 3.17. Enamel defect on mandibular first molar caused by attrition.

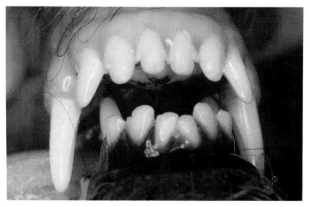

Fig. 3.18. Base narrow canines.

C/H—calculus heavy

C/mod—calculus moderate

C/sl—calculus slight

CA—carious lesion. Craterlike lesion also called a cavity. Occurs mainly in the molar pits of large dogs (Fig. 3.19).

C—craze lines. Abnormal stress on enamel surface forms small cracks on crown (Fig. 3.20).

CR—crowding (Fig. 3.21).

D—dehiscence. Absence of bone support around root (Fig. 3.22).

E—enamel defect (Fig. 3.23).

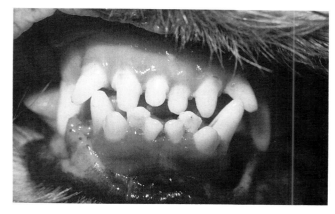

Fig. 3.21. Crowding of mandibular incisor teeth in Shih Tzu.

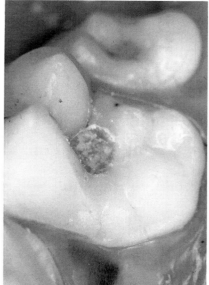

Fig. 3.19. Carious lesion in pit of first molar.

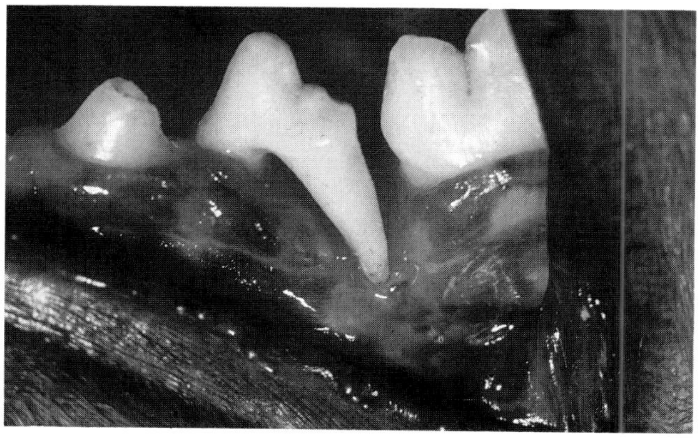

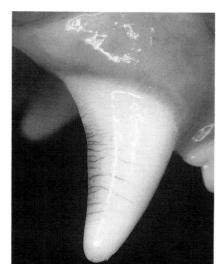

Fig. 3.20. Craze lines on maxillary canine.

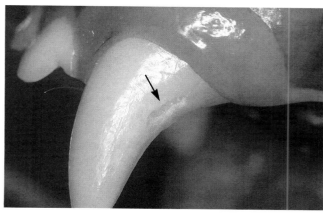

Fig. 3.22. Dehiscence.

Fig. 3.23. Enamel defect (arrow).

EH—enamel hypoplasia. A condition where enamel is thin or absent (Fig. 3.24). Appears as areas of shiny enamel surrounded by opaque areas of dentin. In time, the opaque regions become stained a brownish color. In dogs, enamel hypoplasia is usually caused by a febrile disease, occurring as the enamel is forming before the animal is six months old.

EP—epulis. A periodontal growth classified as either fibromatous, ossifying, or acanthomatous (Figs. 3.25 and 3.26).

ER—external resorption. Loss of tooth substance from outside influences such as cementoclastic and dentoclastic action (Fig. 3.27).

X—extracted tooth.

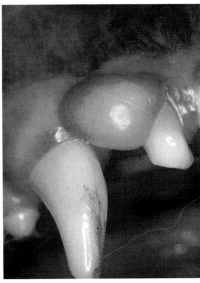

Fig. 3.25. Fibromatous epulis.

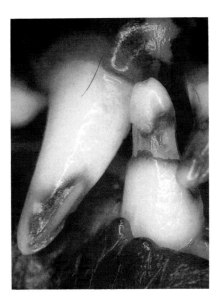

Fig. 3.24. Enamel hypoplasia.

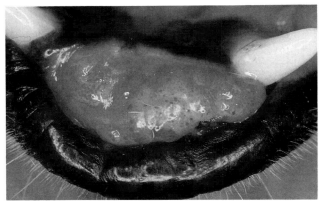

Fig. 3.26. Locally expanding acanthomatous epulis.

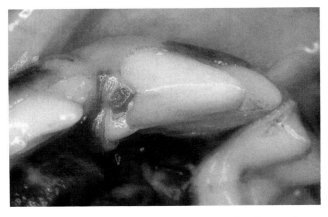

Fig. 3.27. External resorption lesion on maxillary fourth premolar.

Fen—fenestration. A round or oval defect or opening in the alveolar cortical plate of bone over the root surface (Fig. 3.28).

FX—fractured tooth

FGG—free gingival graft. Transplanting attached gingiva from one area of the mouth to another.

FWS—freeway space. The space between the maxillary and mandibular premolar opposing teeth cusp tips when the mouth is closed.

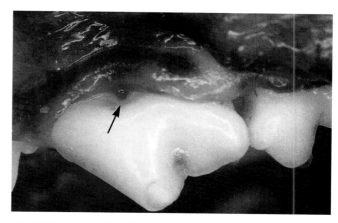

Fig. 3.29. Incipient furcation exposure (arrow).

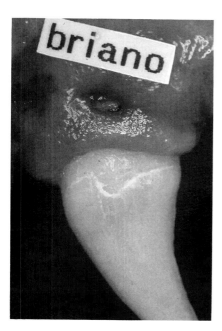

Fig. 3.28. Fenestration.

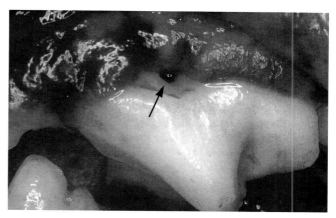

Fig. 3.30. Definite furcation exposure in dog (arrow).

F—furcation exposure

• F1—Class 1 (incipient) furcation exposure exists when the tip of a probe can enter just 1 mm into the furcation area. Bone fills most of the area where the roots meet (Fig. 3.29).

• F2—Class 2 (definite) furcation exposure exists when the probe tip extends more than 1 mm horizontally into the area where the roots converge (Fig. 3.30).

• F3—Class 3 (through and through) furcation exposure exists when the alveolar bone has eroded to a point that the explorer probe passes through the defect unobstructed (Fig. 3.31).

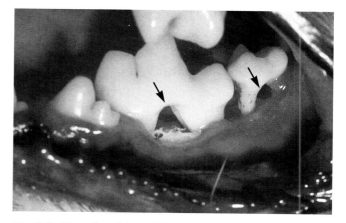

Fig. 3.31. Through and through furcation exposure in dog (arrows).

FU—fusion. Union of two teeth buds. The root canals may be separate or joined. Clinically, there is one less tooth in the arch. Radiographically, there will be two roots with one crown (Fig. 3.32).

GE—gemination. The division of a single tooth at the time of development resulting in incomplete formation of two teeth (Figs. 3.33 and 3.34). On radiographs there will be one root with a split crown. Clinically, there will be an extra tooth in the arch.

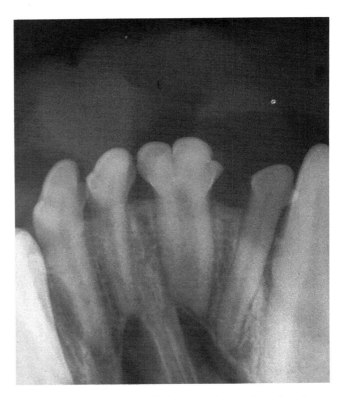

Fig. 3.32. Fusion of two tooth buds. Notice decreased number of incisors in maxilla.

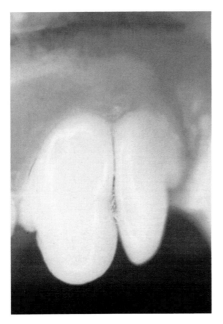

Fig. 3.33.
Gemination of one tooth with two crowns.

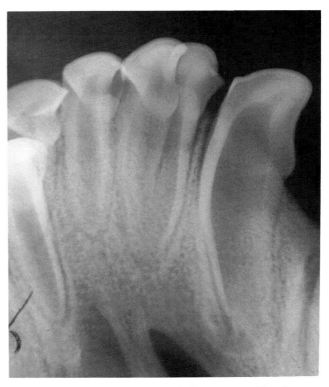

Fig. 3.34. Radiograph confirming teeth share one root. Note three incisor roots and four crowns on right side of maxilla.

H—gingival hyperplasia. Proliferation of attached gingiva coronal to the cemento-enamel junction (Fig. 3.35).

GR—gingival recession. Areas where the gingival margin exists apical to the cemento-enamel junction (CEJ) (Fig. 3.36).

GV—gingivectomy

I—impacted tooth. A tooth that cannot erupt or complete its eruption due to its contact with an obstruction.

LB—level bite. Where the maxillary and mandibular incisors meet at the incisal edges (Fig. 3.37).

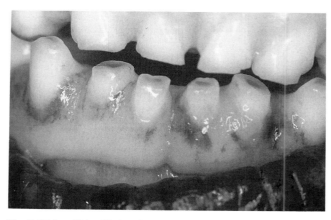

Fig. 3.37. Level bite. Notice abnormal incisal wear.

O—missing tooth. Adult dogs normally have 42 teeth, cats 30. Missing teeth occur for various reasons (Figs. 3.38 and 3.39):

- Congenital absence
- Impaction of an unerupted tooth
- Previous trauma causing exfoliation or fracture
- Previous dental care

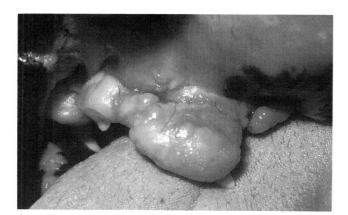

Fig. 3.35. Gingival hyperplasia.

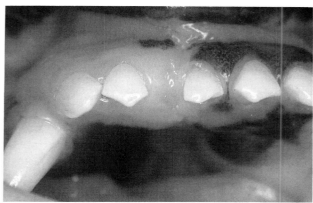

Fig. 3.38. Missing right maxillary central incisor. Radiographs must be taken to check etiology.

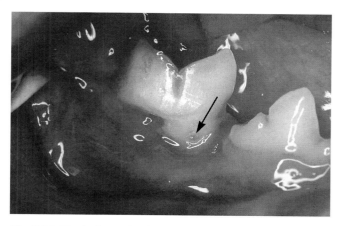

Fig. 3.36. Gingival recession (arrow).

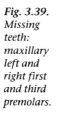

Fig. 3.39. Missing teeth: maxillary left and right first and third premolars.

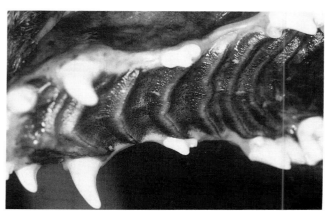

Used to evaluate the cause of missing teeth, radiographs reveal if there is an impacted tooth, retained or fractured root, or no root.

M—mobile tooth. An important diagnostic sign that results from a decrease in root attachment or changes in the periodontal ligament. Mobility is noted as M1, M2, and M3 based on severity.

NE—near exposure. Fractured tooth with near pulpal exposure.

N—neck lesion. Feline odontoclastic resorptive lesion (FORL).

- Class 1—Enamel or cementum loss only
- Class 2—Enamel and dentin exposure (Fig. 3.40)
- Class 3—Pulpal exposure (Fig. 3.41)
- Class 4—Partial crown loss (Fig. 3.42)
- Class 5—Full crown loss (Fig. 3.43)

OD—odontoplasty. Area of tooth reshaped by dental bur.

OB—open bite. An abnormal area of open space when the jaw is closed. It normally should be occupied by occluding teeth.

OM—oral mass

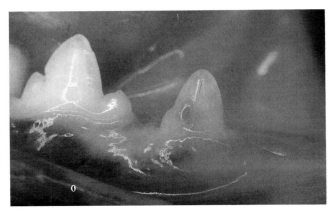

Fig. 3.40. Class 2 FORL.

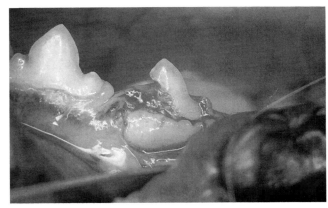

Fig. 3.42. Class 4 FORL.

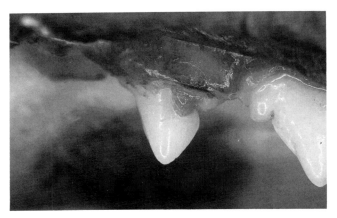

Fig. 3.41. Class 3 FORL.

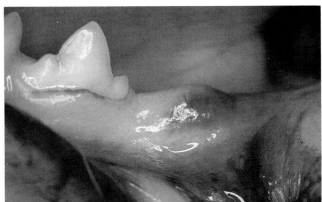

Fig. 3.43. Class 5 FORL.

ONF—oronasal fistula. An abnormal communication between the mouth and nasal cavity (Fig. 3.44).

PP—periodontal pocket—Loss of gingival attachment (Fig. 3.45).

PCB—posterior crossbite. A malocclusion where one or more of the mandibular premolar teeth occlude buccally with the maxillary teeth (Fig. 3.46).

PE—pulpal exposure. Opening of the pulp canal, exposing blood vessels, nerves, and cellular elements to the outside environment. Usually caused by trauma (Fig. 3.47).

PU—pulpitis. Inflammation of the pulp results in discoloration of the tooth (Fig. 3.48).

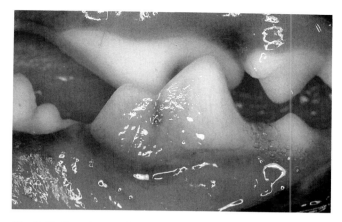

Fig. 3.46. Posterior crossbite. The maxillary fourth premolar is located palatal rather than buccal to mandibular first molar.

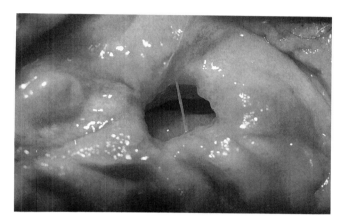

Fig. 3.44. Oronasal fistula.

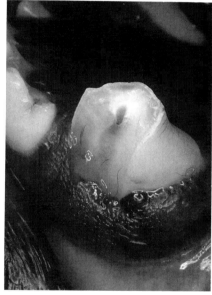

Fig. 3.47. Pulpal exposure from fractured tooth.

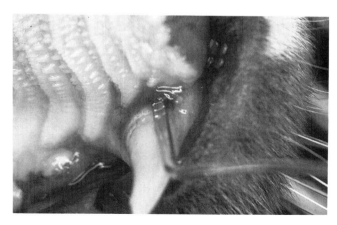

Fig. 3.45. Eight-mm palatal periodontal pocket in a cat's canine.

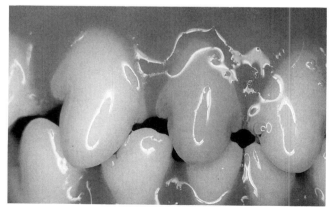

Fig. 3.48. Pulpitis. Compare the discolored tooth with those adjacent.

3D—reparative or sclerotic dentin. Shiny, transparent dentin formed as a defense mechanism to chronic irritation (Fig. 3.49).

R/A—restoration/amalgam (Fig. 3.50)

R/C—restoration/composite (Fig. 3.51)

R/I—restoration/glass ionomer

R/M—restoration/metallic crown (Fig. 3.52)

RD—retained deciduous teeth. Primary teeth that have not been shed when secondary (permanent) teeth erupt (Fig. 3.53).

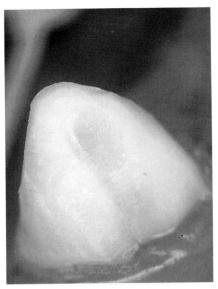

Fig. 3.51. Composite restoration.

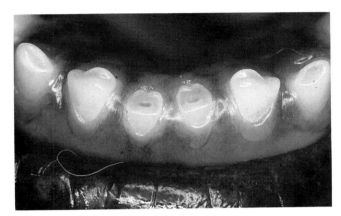

Fig. 3.49. Shiny sclerotic dentin.

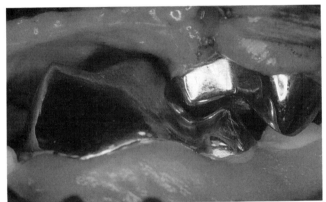

Fig. 3.52. Metallic crowns restoring function to fractured teeth.

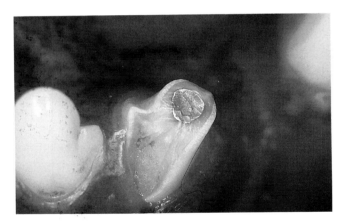

Fig. 3.50. Amalgam restoration.

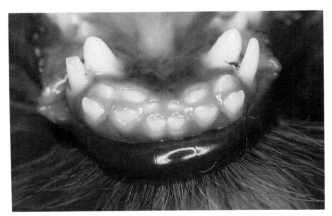

Fig. 3.53. Retained mandibular deciduous canine and incisor teeth displacing adult teeth to abnormal locations.

RR—retained root. Areas where crown is no longer apparent but root(s) remain (Figs. 3.54–3.56).

RCT—root canal therapy

RPC—root planing, closed

RPO—root planing, open

R—rotated. A rotated tooth is usually secondary to tooth crowding. Most commonly affected teeth are the maxillary second and third premolars (Fig. 3.57).

SE—supereruption. Condition where the cemento-enamel junction of a tooth is erupted more coronal than normal. Most common in the canines of older cats (Fig. 3.58).

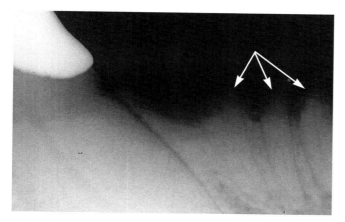

Fig. 3.54. Radiograph of retained roots (arrows).

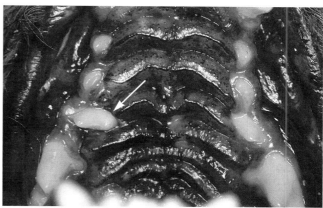

Fig. 3.57. Rotated maxillary third premolar (arrow).

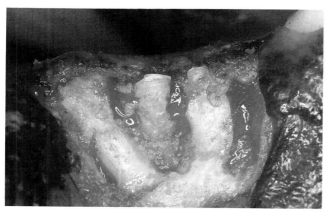

Fig. 3.55. Flap surgery for retained roots.

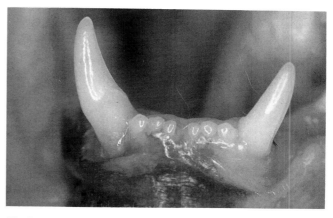

Fig. 3.58. Supererupted mandibular canine tooth in a cat.

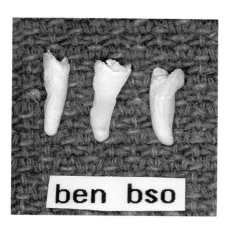

Fig. 3.56. Extraction of retained roots.

S—supernumerary tooth. Extra adult tooth in the arch. Most commonly located in the incisor and premolar areas (Figs. 3.59 and 3.60). Supernumerary teeth may cause overcrowding, leading to periodontal disease or traumatic occlusion.

V—vital pulpotomy. Surgical amputation of a portion of the dental pulp and restoration of the reduced crown resulting in a vital tooth.

WF—wear facet. A flattened, highly polished area on the tooth's surface from chronic wear (Fig. 3.61).

W—worn tooth. Usually a tooth subject to abrasion from grinding or wearing away of tooth substance by mastication (Fig. 3.62).

WB—wry bite or wry mouth. A skeletal defect where the midline of the maxilla does not line up with the midline of the mandible (Fig. 3.63).

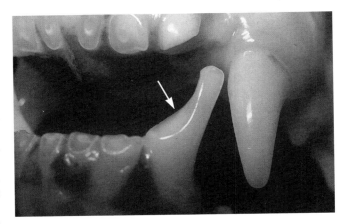

Fig. 3.61. Wear facet from attrition (arrow).

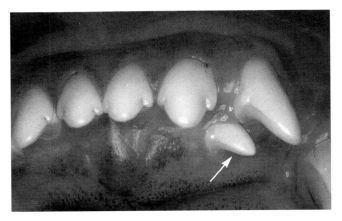

Fig. 3.59. Supernumerary lateral incisor tooth (arrow).

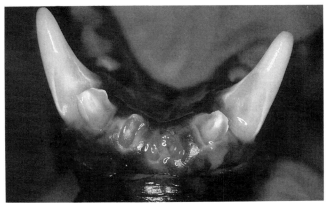

Fig. 3.62. Teeth abraided from chewing on hair coat.

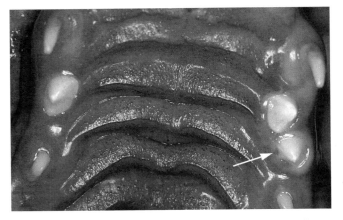

Fig. 3.60. Extra maxillary first premolar (arrow). *Extraction will prevent overcrowding.*

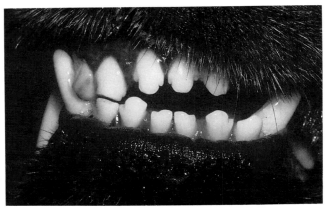

Fig. 3.63. Wry bite. Notice triangular defect in the incisor area.

INDICES USED TO RECORD ORAL HEALTH

The **Periodontal Index (PDI)** measures the incidence and severity of periodontal disease. Scores, ranging from 0 to 4, measure soft tissue inflammation and loss of periodontal support as indicated by radiographs and mobility.

The **Oklahoma Canine Oral Health Index** can also be used to evaluate periodontal health. A record is made of gingival inflammation, calculus, plaque, probing depth, and attachment level. Four maxillary (left lateral, left canine, left fourth premolar, and left first molar) and four mandibular (left canine, left second premolar, left fourth premolar, and left first molar) teeth are evaluated and the results recorded.

The **Gingival Index (GI)** grades the severity of buccal gingival inflammation.

0=No inflammation
1=Mild inflammation—Marginal redness only, no bleeding on probing
2=Moderate inflammation—Increased redness, pinpoint bleeding upon gentle probing, edema. Gingiva is red, swollen, and bleeds on gentle probing of sulcus.
3=Severe inflammation—Red or blue-red gingiva, purulent exudate, evidence of tissue necrosis, spontaneous bleeding

For the **Calculus Index (CI)** teeth are gently air-dried and evaluated buccally.

0=No calculus
1=Calculus covering less than one-half of clinical crown
2=Calculus covering more than one-half of clinical crown
3=Gingival recession with calculus present on root surface

Feline and canine dental calculus will often **fluoresce** under a Wood's ultraviolet light. Using this technique will help convince some clients that their pets' teeth need to be professionally cleaned.

Red fluorescence seen under the ultraviolet light is due to porphyrins produced by bacteria. Once the dog or cat has its teeth cleaned and polished, fluorescence disappears.

For the **Plaque Index**, teeth are evaluated by applying disclosing solution to the buccal surface of each tooth and immediately rinsing with water.

0=No plaque
1=Separate flecks of plaque
2=Plaque covering less than one-third of crown
3=Plaque covering at least one-third, but less than two-thirds, of crown
4=Plaque covering two-thirds or more of crown

ORAL EXFOLIATIVE CYTOLOGY

Often lesions are discovered in the mouth that are caused by neoplasia. Using cytology (the examination of cells), the veterinarian may be able to differentiate between infection, inflammation, and malignancy. Cell examination is a rapid way to "get a handle" on the cause of pathology, but it does not replace the specificity of biopsy.

Instruments required for cytology are minimal, consisting of

- A cotton swab
- A 6-cc syringe with 18-gauge needle
- A standard microscope slide
- Diff Quick stain

Cells can be harvested and placed upon a microscopic slide for examination through one of the following:

- Smearing the lesion with a cotton swab. This is commonly used where ulcerated lesions are present.

- Scraping the lesion with a moistened tongue blade or cement spatula

- Placing the slide against the lesion (touch impression). This is rarely used in the oral cavity due to accessibility. It may be used on facial lesions.

- Obtaining cells via needle aspiration of solid masses

Cytodiagnosis: What to Look for under the Microscope

The criteria of **malignancy** are based on changes in structure of individual cells (Figs. 3.64–3.66). The nucleus holds most of the diagnostic clues.

Nuclear changes consistent with malignancy:

- Disproportionate enlargement of the nucleus
- Decrease in the cell/nucleus ratio

- Hyperchromasia
- Enlarged nucleoli
- Multinucleation
- Abundant mitotic figures
- Pleomorphism

The **interrelationship of cells** is also important to examine. Lack of cell boundaries, the grouping and crowding of cells, and the engulfing of one cell by another are also indicators of malignancy.

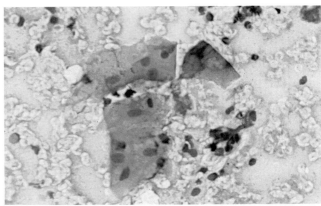

Fig. 3.66. Benign squamous epithelial cells from the surface of an epulis. Cells are polygonal with small nuclei. Note the low nuclear to cytoplasmic ratio. Compare the size of the nucleus with the inflammatory cells and red blood cells in the background. Cells may detach in small clusters, but clusters have smooth outlines. The total number of epithelial cells and cell clusters on the smear is low. (400x)

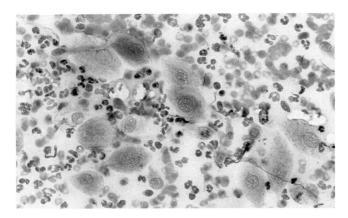

Fig. 3.64. Cytology of squamous cell carcinoma. The smear is cellular with many cell clusters. Cell clusters have irregular outlines. Individual cells have large, dark nuclei, prominent nucleoli, and high nuclear to cytoplasmic ratios. Compare the size of the nucleus with the inflammatory cells and red blood cells in the background. Individual cells have a tendency to form elongated, spindled shapes. (400x)

SUMMARY

Only a thorough and exacting examination of the patient's teeth, periodontium, soft tissue, and occlusion provides adequate information for a diagnosis. After abnormalities of the structures are radiographed, diagnosed, and recorded, the treatment planning process begins. A treatment plan and subsequent therapy are only as effective as the quality of information obtained during the examination.

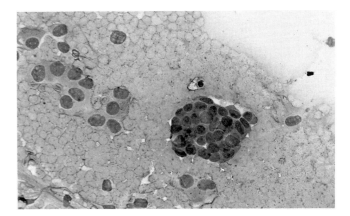

Fig. 3.65. Cytology of malignant cells from an adenocarcinoma. The smear is cellular with many hyperchromatic cell clusters. Cell clusters have irregular outlines. This cell cluster forms an acinus or gland with a central lumen. Individual cells have large, dark nuclei, prominent nucleoli, and high nuclear to cytoplasmic ratios. Individual cells tend to maintain ovoid shapes and do not generally have the elongated, spindled shapes of squamous cell carcinoma. Compare these cells with the squamous cell carcinoma (Fig. 3.64). (200x)

4. EQUIPPING YOUR DENTAL PRACTICE

Begin; to begin is half the work. Let half still remain;
again begin this, and thou wilt have finished.
—AUSONIUS

Acquiring the proper equipment and staff to perform dentistry is one of the wisest investments a practitioner can make. There is no other branch of small animal medicine where a relatively minimal financial investment can provide such patient and practice benefit.

When faced with equipping your dental practice, envision the level of involvement you wish to achieve in the various aspects of veterinary dentistry; then acquire the equipment and education necessary to practice at that level. Leaving room for growth, it is better to overplan than to underplan.

THREE LEVELS OF DENTAL EQUIPMENT

For $10,000–15,000 you can purchase most everything necessary to provide the best in dentistry. Not a high figure when you realize that the return on the investment is immediate and continuous. For instance, without a dental radiograph unit, you cannot diagnose greater than 60 percent of the oral pathology hiding below the gingiva.

You may want to set your dental equipment sights on three levels, from basic to advanced.

Level One:
Basic Examination and Teeth Cleaning

Equipment needs:

- Mouth prop
- Charts for dental examination findings
- Explorer probe
- Periodontal probe
- Oral mirror
- Radiograph film (sizes 0, 2, 4) for use with standard radiograph machine

- Chairside developer
- Rapid developer and fixer chemicals
- Curettes
- Luxators
- Extraction forceps
- Root tip pick
- Eye and respiratory protection devices
- Ultrasonic scaler and polisher, with at least two types of tips (gross scaling-spatula and fine point periodontal/interproximal tip)
- Fluoride
- Polishing materials
- Home care products and promotional materials

Estimated cost: $2000–3000.

Level Two:
Extractions and Minor Periodontal Surgery

- Periosteal elevators (Molt, Freer)
- High-speed/low-speed delivery system, with assortment of cutting instruments (round, inverted, fissure burs)
- Dental radiograph unit

Estimated cost in addition to level one is $5000–6500 (including the high-speed delivery system).

Level Three:
Endodontics, Comprehensive Periodontal Surgery, Orthodontics, Restoration, and Oral Surgery

- Endodontic materials

  — Assortment of round burs
  — Kerr files 21–30 mm long from sizes 8 to 60
  — Hedstrom files 60 mm long, sizes 10–80

— Barbed broaches
— Twenty-seven-gauge blunted endodontic needle
— Sodium hypochlorite solution
— Mixing slab
— Mixing spatula
— Gutta-percha in multiple lengths and widths
— Spreader (small, medium, and large)
— Plugger (small, medium, and large)
— Paper points
— Zinc oxide-eugenol

• **Restorative materials**

— Etching gel
— Bonding resin and brush
— Unfilled, filled, and hybrid restoratives
— Plastic matrix strips
— Curing light
— Finishing kit
— Abrasive strips
— Polishing kit
— Rubber-based impression material

• **Orthodontic equipment**

— Alginate
— Mouth molds
— Boxing wax
— Plaster
— Bracket cement
— Elastics

Estimated cost in addition to levels one and two: $2000–3000.

Plan B

Often dental equipment does not function properly. Having backup delivery systems, light-curing wands, and high- and low-speed handpieces proves invaluable.

THE DENTAL OPERATORY

Creating the ideal place to practice dentistry is challenging. Unfortunately, by the time most practitioners realize they want to make dentistry a major part of their practices, the facilities have already been built without sufficient space for comfortable dental care delivery. Fortunately, dental equipment is compact and can be adapted to fit a majority of practices (Fig. 4.1).

The challenge is to provide a safe area to use and store dental supplies, the delivery system, the dental radiograph unit, the radiograph developer, the suction device, illumination, general anesthesia, and monitoring equipment. Wall-mounted equipment is preferable to floor-based.

A 12- by 15-ft area is ideal for dental therapy. Space for at least two tables should be planned. The dental operatory must not be located in the same room where general surgery is performed. Bacteria-laden aerosols released during ultrasonic scaling may contaminate the room. Many practices perform dental procedures in the treatment area. Although this works, it is not ideal. So much activity is going on in the treatment room that the operator cannot concentrate on the dental patient.

It is best to plan a stand-alone dental operatory, where everything related to dentistry is in one easily accessible area. Some measurements:

• The ideal operatory table is 7 ft long and 2$^{1}/_{2}$ ft wide.

• The working end of the table is between 36 and 38 in. high with adequate room beneath the table so that the practitioner's or technician's knees easily fit.

• The table should be slanted toward a drain.

Dental procedures are best performed sitting down. An adjustable stool with rollers is helpful.

Utilities needed include electricity, water, and drainage. Multiple electrical grounded outlets (at least eight) are recommended to help power the delivery system, light cure gun, amalgamator, light source, radiograph viewer, monitoring equipment, and heating pad.

Water is used in the high-speed delivery system to cool heat generated by drilling. If the water in your area contains an abundance of minerals, a filter is recommended to decrease sediment collected. Distilled water can be held in a stand-alone unit where water is poured into a holding tank.

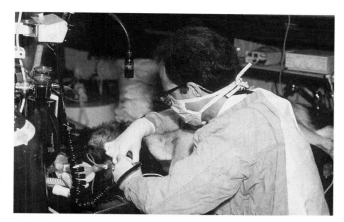

Fig. 4.1. Dental operatory.

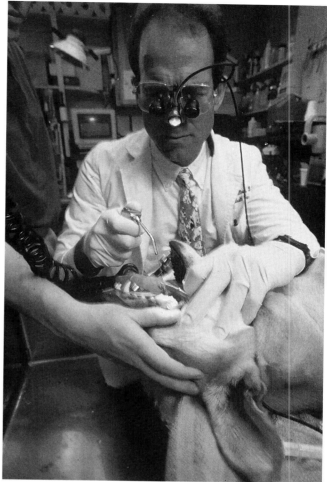

Fig. 4.2. Orascoptic Research headlamp provides an intense light source magnification.

Storage of equipment and materials requires careful organization. When hand instruments, power equipment, and dental materials are jumbled in a drawer, confusion, wasted time, and poorly sterilized instruments are the result.

At least two locations are used for storage. For primary storage, a cabinet or set of drawers within easy reach of the operator is utilized to store frequently used instruments and materials. A secondary location can be utilized to stockpile resupply items.

Storage drawers are arranged by dental procedure. The periodontal drawer contains sterilized packs of hand instruments and supplies for performing gingival examinations and surgery. Likewise for the endodontic, oral surgical, restorative, and orthodontic compartments. Oversized drawers are used for larger pieces of equipment and supplies. The key is to have all necessary supplies within easy reach.

Lighting and magnification are fundamental for the practice of dentistry. A spotlight is necessary to illuminate the oral cavity. Spotlights come in different configurations. Ceiling-mounted or wall-mounted light sources are maneuverable and out of the way. Floor-mounted spotlights work well but can be cumbersome and take up valuable floor space. Additionally, high-speed handpieces can be equipped with fiber-optic light sources to illuminate the field. Head-mounted spotlights accompanied with magnifying telescopes enhance the lighting of the working environment (Fig. 4.2).

High-speed dental delivery systems are fundamental in the dental operatory (Figs. 4.4–4.10). Compressed air– or gas-powered units control the drills, sonic cleaners, suction, and water. Needle valves regulate water

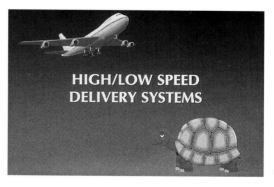

Fig. 4.3.

and air flow. "Silent" refrigerator compressors can be contained at the delivery unit. Larger compressors are located remotely to minimize noise. Wherever your compressor is placed, easy access is essential to provide maintenance and repair.

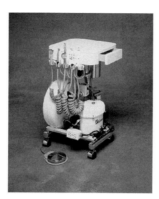

Fig. 4.4. Henry Schein Vet Base 5 dental delivery system.

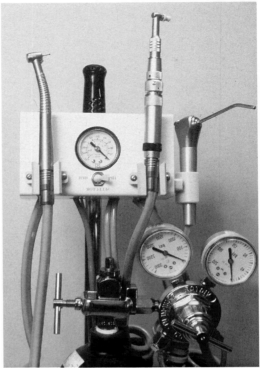

Fig. 4.6. Cbi Nitair dental delivery system, powered by nitrogen.

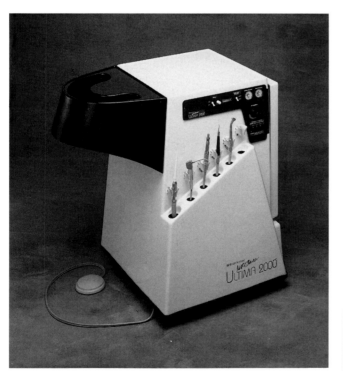

Fig. 4.5. Henry Schein Ultima 2000 dental delivery system.

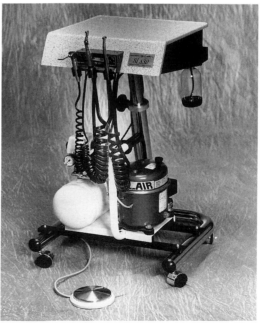

Fig. 4.7. Sage-London Industries SL830 veterinary dental delivery system.

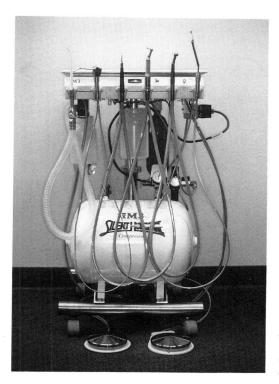

Fig. 4.8.
iM3 dental
delivery
system.

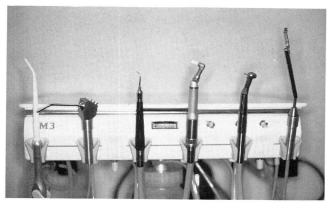

Fig. 4.9. Handpiece options on the iM3 dental delivery system:
(from left) suction, water/air spray, sonic scaler, low-speed handpiece
with polishing angle, high-speed handpiece, fiber-optic light.

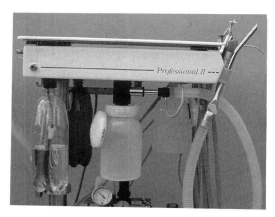

Fig. 4.10.
Suction
and
irrigation
bottle on
iM3
delivery
system.

Radiography is fundamental to performing veterinary dentistry. Human patients help their doctors diagnose pathology by expressing feelings of pain, temperature, or pressure. Even with this help, dentists need radiographs to evaluate the extent of dental lesions.

Because veterinary patients cannot speak, the dental radiograph unit must be used to evaluate dental structures. *Radiography is the most useful diagnostic aid available to the veterinarian practicing dentistry.* While dental radiographs may be taken with the standard whole body machine, its location and fixed nature require animal patients to be moved from the dental table to the radiograph area. With endodontic procedures, patient relocation would have to be performed multiple times, which adds time and inconvenience to the operation. The dedicated dental radiograph unit is an essential piece of equipment in the dental operatory.

The radiograph unit can be purchased with a retractable tube arm extending up to 6 ft. The long arm helps tube positioning regardless of where the patient's head is. Controls can be wall, table, ceiling, or floor mounted. Dental units operate on 110 volts and require separate 30-amp circuits. They cost between $2500 and $4000.

ANESTHESIA NEEDS

By necessity, dentistry is performed while the small animal is anesthetized. This allows the practitioner and technician to perform procedures on immobilized patients without causing pain. Incorporating anesthetic delivery systems in the operatory console increases efficiency.

Patient-monitoring devices are helpful for the safe delivery of anesthesia. Some dental procedures require hours of anesthesia. In addition, many small animal patients with periodontal disease are older and may become compromised under anesthesia. Electrocardiograph monitoring, pulse oximeters, respiratory alarms, end tidal carbon dioxide, and constant blood pressure observation add to the safety of performing anesthesia on dental patients (Figs. 4.11–4.14).

Hypercarbia (elevated carbon dioxide) and hypoxemia (low blood oxygen) result from inadequate ventilation and are potential complications in anesthetized animals. Virtually all anesthetic medication depresses ventilation. Visually, the effects on ventilation can be monitored by mucus membrane color and the depth and number of respiratory efforts. Unfortunately, with shallow respiratory efforts, an animal can be hypoventilating and still appear to have normal appearing gingiva.

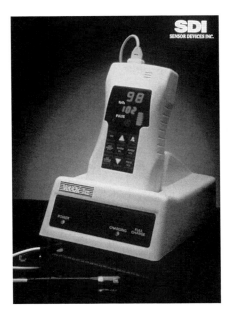

Fig. 4.11. Pulse oximeter. Courtesy of SDI Company.

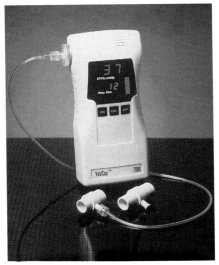

Fig. 4.13. End tidal carbon dioxide monitor. Courtesy of SDI Company.

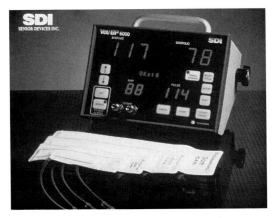

Fig. 4.12. Blood pressure monitor. Courtesy of SDI Company.

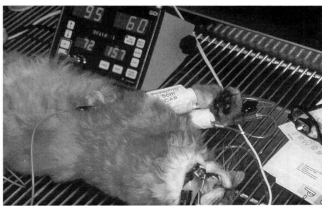

Fig. 4.14. Patient under anesthesia with monitor equipment attached.

The use of the pulse oximeter and capnometer has changed subjective anesthesia monitoring to objective monitoring "by the numbers."

- **Pulse oximeters** measure hemoglobin saturation with oxygen through the attachment of a monitor probe on the tongue, toe pad, pinna, vulva, or tail. Normal oxygen readings are greater than 95 percent.

- **Capnometry** measures the buildup of carbon dioxide. Normal readings are between 35 and 45 mmHg. If higher than 45 mm Hg, the patient is hypoventilating and retaining carbon dioxide. Decreasing the anesthetic and/or assisting ventilation would be indicated. Lower readings may indicate hyperventilation.

POWER EQUIPMENT

Power equipment is necessary to perform dentistry efficiently. Teeth may be scaled using only hand instruments, but the added time and hand fatigue make hand scaling inefficient. Power is required for polishing, which must be part of every dental cleaning procedure. Most advanced dental procedures cannot be done without power equipment.

Electrical Sonic and Ultrasonic Scalers

When plaque remains on the teeth for only a few days, it mineralizes, creating tartar (calculus). These deposits are hard minerals, which cannot be removed by routine brushing. Scalers are used to remove plaque and tartar from the crown. Scaling can be performed with hand or power instruments. Powered scalers increase the speed and efficiency of cleaning teeth. They are classified as either sonic or ultrasonic.

SONIC SCALERS

Sonic (also called subsonic) scalers are attached to the high-speed outlet of an air- or gas-driven delivery system (Fig. 4.15).

PROS: The tip vibrates at approximately 6 kHz. Due to the low vibration frequency, sonic scalers, when used subgingivally, cause less gingival and pulpal damage than ultrasonic units, but remove too much cementum. Water is not required to cool the tip but is recommended to wash away debris.

Cons: Sonic scalers are weak and may stall out when pressed against a tooth. The sonic scaler unit requires continuous air pressure of 40 psi. A relatively large compressor (greater than 1 hp) is needed for power. Also, due to the low vibration frequency, it may take more time to clean teeth, and more damage may be done to the enamel and cementum surfaces. If the delivery system is oxygen, nitrogen, or carbon dioxide driven, use of sonic scalers can consume large volumes of gas, which may not be economically feasible. Daily lubrication is necessary for maintenance. Additionally, sonic scalers break down more often.

ULTRASONIC SCALERS

Ultrasonic scalers vibrate at 18–42 kHz, converting sound waves into mechanical vibration. Water, energized as it passes over the vibrating tip, produces a scouring effect to remove plaque, calculus, and some stains. Electric ultrasonic scalers are classified as magnetorestrictive or piezoelectric. The scaler fractures calculus when a light sweeping stroke across the tooth is made with the tip's side. Water mist cools the tip and flushes away debris. Most ultrasonic scalers must not be used subgingivally because of thermal damage that can injure the gingival sulcus and pulp. (The Odontoson by Periogene is designed to be used subgingivally without damaging these tissues. Thin-Line and Slim-Line tips made by Dentsply and Hu-Friedy Company may be used subgingivally.)

PROS: The ultrasonic scaler cycles between 20 and 42 kHz, generating considerable scaling power.

Cons: With most ultrasonic units (other than the Odontoson), heat at the tip can cause damage, so the tip should not be placed below the gum line. Pulpal damage resulting in tooth death can occur if the point is allowed to remain in contact with the tooth for more than a few seconds. In time the tip becomes dull and needs replacement.

Magnetorestrictive scalers use an insert (called a **stack**) made of strips of laminated nickel that vibrate, causing the tip to move in an elliptical pattern. These strips vibrate at up to 30 kHz (Figs. 4.16 and 4.17).

Recently, the **Odontoson**, a high-frequency magnetorestrictive ultrasonic unit, was introduced to the dental profession (Figs. 4.18 and 4.19). The Odontoson utilizes a ferric rod that generates less heat compared with

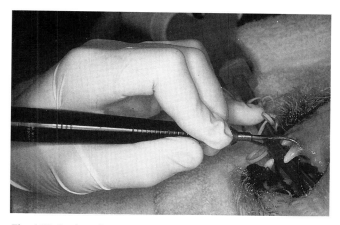

Fig. 4.15. Sonic scaler.

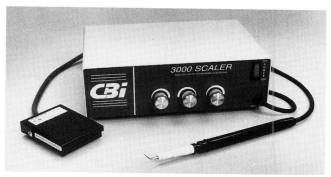

Fig. 4.17. Cbi magnetorestrictive scaler.

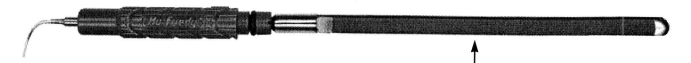

Fig. 4.16. Magnetorestrictive scaler and stack (arrow).

the conventional metal stack used in other ultrasonic units. The special slim titanium tip moves in a rotational pattern at a high frequency (up to 42 kHz) at low amplitude and can be used subgingivally.

Piezoelectric scalers have two quartz crystals that expand and contract at a constant frequency when electrical energy is supplied to the transducer.

Pros: Piezoelectric scalers oscillate at 30-40 kHz. The tip is screwed into a metal base attached rigidly to the crystals. Replacing the tip is less expensive than replacing a magnetorestrictive stack. The tip vibrates in a linear fashion much like hand scaling. Less heat is generated with the piezoelectric scaler.

Cons: The piezoelectric tip can generate an aggressive vibration that may cause enamel damage. Vibration energy in the tip is not distributed evenly. The most active side should be placed against calculus to be removed. One hundred and ten volts are used to energize the crystals in the handle. Used in the presence of water, the piezoelectric scaler may create an electrical hazard.

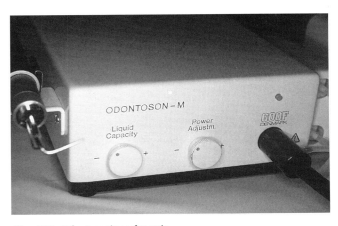

Fig. 4.18. Odontosonic scaler unit.

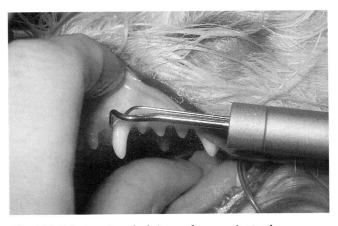

Fig. 4.19. Odontosonic scaler being used on a canine tooth.

Rotosonic scalers use a six-sided stainless steel bur that rotates in the high-speed handpiece at speeds over 300,000 rpm (Fig. 4.20). When applied to the tooth surfaces, the bur shatters calculus, which is flushed away by cooling water.

Pros: None.

Cons: Depending on the operator, when removing calculus, the rotosonic bur may chip enamel, exposing dentin. Additionally, rotosonic burs are thick (even the periodontal flame points), and unless used by an experienced operator, the burs may damage sulcular tissue. Lastly, the rotosonic bur dulls readily and must be replaced often.

SCALER INSERTS

The *side* of the scaler insert is the operative part of the scaler. *Do not use the tip's end on the tooth or periodontal tissues.*

Modified periodontal inserts are slender tips resembling periodontal probes; this similarity makes access to tight interproximal and diseased furcation areas easier for periodontal debridement (Figs. 4.21 and 4.22). The goal when using periodontal Slim-Line or Thin-Line tips is to disrupt bacterial plaque rather than to remove cementum. To perform "microultrasonic scaling":

- Use increased water flow for irrigation.

- Set power 75 percent lower than usual to avoid overheating and patient or instrument harm.

- Work with a light touch.

- Imagine that you are using an eraser to remove pencil markings or a crayon to fill space between lines. Move the tip across the root surface in a definite pattern of overlapping strokes.

- Subgingivally, keep the tip in constant motion.

Clinical studies on humans show patient benefits from periodontal treatment provided by the modified inserts exceed those from hand instrumentation. Modified periodontal tips in an ultrasonic device have been shown to produce smoother root surfaces and, when compared with conventional ultrasonics or hand instrumentation, to provide better penetration to the bottom of the pocket. Use of modified periodontal tips may decrease the need for using hand instruments in teeth cleaning.

Beaver tail (spatula) **tips** are broad-based, flat scaler tips routinely used to remove gross calculus (Fig. 4.23).

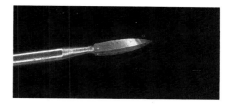

Fig. 4.20. Rotosonic bur.

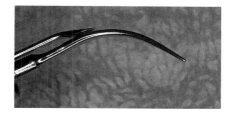

Fig. 4.21. Ultrasonic periodontal tip (Hu-Friedy Company).

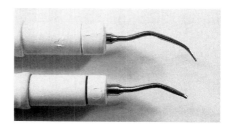

Fig. 4.22. The normal ultrasonic scaler tip (top) and a fractured tip (bottom).

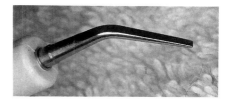

Fig. 4.23. Beaver tail tip ultrasonic insert.

Dental Delivery Units

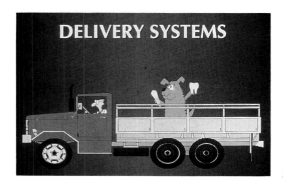

Fig. 4.24.

ELECTRICALLY DRIVEN UNITS

Pros: A portable electric dental micromotor with handpiece is an economical entry-level instrument (Fig. 4.25). A micromotor is used to power the burs, disks, or cups. This unit accepts straight, contra-angle, and prophy angle handpieces.

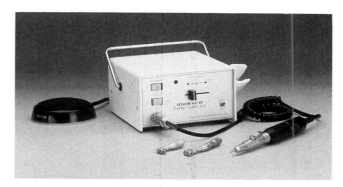

Fig. 4.25. Electric micromotor.

Cons: The electric unit is limited without compressed air to dry the teeth for restorative procedures and without water for cooling. If an electric micromotor is used, an assistant must spray water on the field. Electric units operate below 30,000 rpm at high torque and vibrate, making precise work difficult.

COMPRESSED AIR– AND GAS-DRIVEN UNITS

Compressed air– or gas-driven units are used to facilitate tooth extraction, periodontal surgery, oral surgery, polishing, and endodontics (Fig. 4.26). Their advantage over motorized systems lies in their ability to offer precise cutting and water to cool the high-speed drill. Water prevents thermal damage to the pulp and surrounding bone.

There are two types of air-powered systems: (1) compressed nitrogen or room air stored in a cylinder or (2) use of a compressor to take room air and compress it to drive handpieces.

The basic self-contained system consists of

- A compressor, which provides compressed air

- A pressure or air tank for storage and slow release

- A liquid-holding container for irrigation and cooling

- An assembly delivery system (also called the control panel) containing an air/water supply syringe and tubing for the handpieces. There is a pressure gauge to monitor air pressure, switches for turning water on and off, a needle valve to adjust water flow, and a switch to change from the high- to the low-speed handpiece (Fig. 4.27).

- The handpieces

- A foot switch for starting and stopping the handpieces

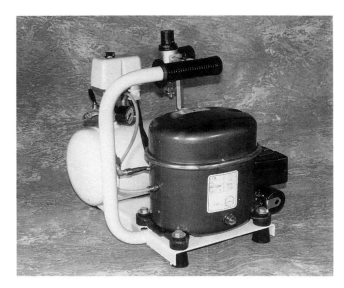

Fig. 4.26. Compressor and air tank.

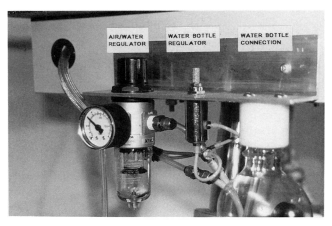

Fig. 4.27. Connections and gauges on delivery system.

The **compressor** must be large enough to maintain a pressure of 30–40 psi at a flow rate of 3 cubic ft per minute. Air compressors are either air- or oil-cooled. Air cooling reduces the amount of contaminants (oil) in the line, but air-driven compressors are noisier and more expensive than oil-cooled.

Modified refrigerator oil–cooled compressors are commonly used in self-contained delivery systems (Fig. 4.28). Make sure you purchase an adequately sized compressor and air tank. If the compressor is too small, it will run almost continuously during use and may overheat. The single-unit compressor is rated at 0.5 hp. If a sonic scaler handpiece is to be used, a double-unit (1 hp) should be considered.

The ideal compressor must be quiet and compact, require low maintenance, and provide a steady source of pressurized, oil- and moisture-free air. Atmospheric air has water vapor that must be removed to provide dry air. Water vapor will accumulate in the compressor and must be periodically drained. Condensation is removed by "bleeding" the cock valve at the bottom of the compressor tank onto a gauze square. There is a dipstick or view port to monitor levels in oil-cooled compressors. Additionally, the air storage tank must be drained weekly to remove condensed water. If this is not done, rust will form rapidly in the tank, leading to failure.

Dental handpieces and **burs** can be compared with industrial power drills and bits used to prepare holes in wood and metal. Low- (slow) and high-speed dental hookups are available on most delivery systems (Fig. 4.9).

The **low-speed handpiece** rotates at 5000–10,000 rpm, contains forward and reverse controls, operates with relatively high torque, and does not use water (Fig. 4.29). It is used for polishing, preparing, and finishing restorations; sectioning teeth for extraction; working with dental models; and operating rotary-driven endodontic files.

Low-speed handpieces may be powered by compressed air or electricity. Adapters are used with the low-speed handpiece so that it may function as a straight handpiece (**SHP**), a contra-angle handpiece (**CAHP**), or a right-angle handpiece (**RAHP**).

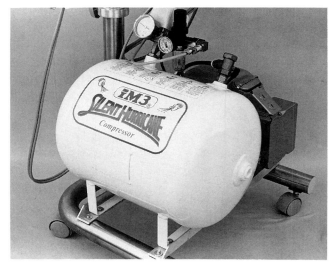

Fig. 4.28. Silent Hurricane compressor from high-/low-speed self-contained delivery system (iM3, Henry Schein, Inc.).

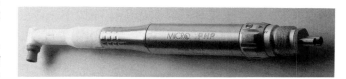

Fig. 4.29. Low-speed handpiece.

• The basic low-speed handpiece is referred to as a **straight handpiece** because of its straight-line design with no bends in the working end. Cutting and polishing instruments that are used in the straight handpiece are designated **HP** (handpiece). An HP designation means that the cutting or polishing instrument has a long, straight shaft that inserts into the straight handpiece.

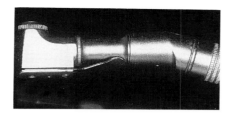

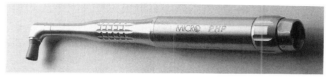

Fig. 4.30. Contra-angle handpiece.

• **Contra-angle handpieces** attach to low-speed straight handpieces to form extensions with angles that are greater than 90 degrees at the working tip (Fig. 4.30). The angulation plus the short shafts of adapted cutting burs provides better access to the posterior teeth. The contra-angle handpiece's main use is for finishing and sanding restorations, slow drilling of root canals with the Gates Glidden drills, filling root canals using Lentulo spiral fillers, and inserting small dental pins for restorations.

Fig. 4.31. Right-angle handpiece.

• **Right-angle handpieces** attach to the low-speed straight handpiece to form an extension with a right angle (90 degrees) at the working tip. The right-angle handpiece (also called the prophy angle) is used to hold polishing cups, disks, and brushes during teeth-cleaning procedures (Figs. 4.31 and 4.32). There are three types of prophylaxis angles:

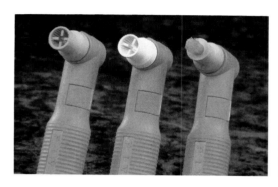

— **Metallic that rotates 360 degrees**—Most commonly used. Easily catches and pulls hair around the animal's lips
— **Metallic that oscillates 90 degrees and reverses**—Will not bother the lip hair
— **Disposable**—Plastic and manufactured for single use

Fig. 4.32. Disposable prophy angles.

There are two ways prophy cups attach to the prophy angles:

— The screw type holds the polishing instrument in place by a threaded shaft.
— The snap-on type has a smooth knob for attachment.

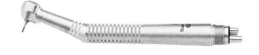

Fig. 4.33. High-speed handpiece.

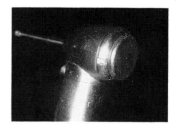

Fig. 4.34. High-speed thumb-operated chuck.

High-speed handpieces are air driven and typically operate at 300,000–400,000 rpm (Fig. 4.33). They are used when the rapid and efficient cutting of the tooth and/or supporting bone is important. To avoid overheating, water is automatically delivered as a spray over the operative field. To ensure better visibility, some high-speed handpieces have a fiber-optic light built into the head. This projects a beam of light from the head of the handpiece directly onto the bur and the tooth undergoing treatment. High-speed handpieces use the friction grip, friction grip surgical, and friction grip short shank burs.

Similar to how an industrial drill bit is secured to the drill, the dental bur is attached to the handpiece with a **chuck** (Fig. 4.34).

• In the low-speed straight handpiece, the chuck is mechanically tightened. After the bur is inserted, the handpiece collar is rotated clockwise to tighten.

• In the low-speed latch-type handpiece, a latch fastens around a notch in the shank of the bur to hold it in place.

• High-speed bur heads are either push button or chuck key style. The bur is placed in the head of the handpiece with a chuck that holds the shank of the bur securely in place by thumb control or with a bur-inserting/removal tool that is used to tighten the chuck clockwise and to remove it counterclockwise.

When purchasing a high-speed handpiece, in order to increase efficiency, buy one that has a thumb-operated chuck.

A **three-way air/water syringe** is part of the high-speed delivery system. The syringe produces a spray or a stream of air or water that rinses debris from the teeth and dries as needed during dental procedures (Fig. 4.35).

BURS: ROTARY CUTTING INSTRUMENTS

Rotary dental instruments are dental handpieces that are used to hold and turn cutting instruments called burs. They have many uses in veterinary dentistry, such as

• Sectioning multirooted teeth to facilitate extraction.
• Providing access points for root canal therapy
• Placement of undercuts for mechanical attachment of bonding material
• Reducing and reshaping teeth for crown preparation
• Polishing teeth

Burs consist of three parts: the shaft, shank, and head.

• The **shaft** is the part of the bur that fits into the handpiece. The length of the shaft depends on the function of the bur. The shape of the shaft is designed to fit into a specific handpiece. Straight handpiece burs (SHP or HP) have a straight shaft usually used in the low-speed handpiece. Latch-type burs have a notch at the opposite end of the bur.

• The **shank** connects the shaft to the head. It is part of the bur that fits into the handpiece. The length of the shank depends on the specific function of the bur. Shanks of surgical burs are longer than those used for restorative finishing. Shank types include the following:

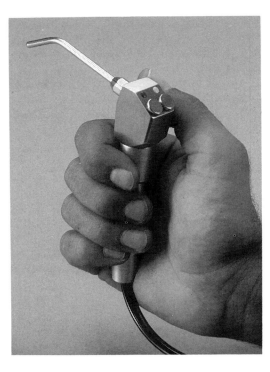

Fig. 4.35. Air/water syringe.

— Straight handpiece burs have long, straight shanks. In catalogs they are abbreviated as **SHP** or **HP**.
— Latch-type burs have notched shanks. In dental catalogs these burs are abbreviated as **LA** (latch-type angle) or **RA** (right-angle).
— Friction grip burs have smooth shanks and are smaller in diameter than HP or RA burs. They are used in high-speed handpieces. Friction grip burs are described as **FG** (friction grip), **FGS** (friction grip surgical), or **FGSS** (friction grip short shank). Surgical burs have longer shanks used to reach into deep recesses while shorter restorative burs are utilized next to the tooth surface.

• The **head** is the cutting end of a bur. Bur types include the following.

— Carbide steel burs are referred to as **carbides**. They are the most commonly used burs.
— Diamond points, referred to as **diamonds**, are burs in which the cutting portion is covered with bits of industrial diamonds (Fig. 4.36). Diamonds are used for crown preparation and shaping teeth. These burs vary in shape and coarseness.
— **Stones**, identified by their color, are used for polishing and finishing restorations. The white stone bur is most commonly used in veterinary dental practice to finish composite restorations (Figs. 4.37 and 4.38). Green abrasive stones are used to finish amalgam and to smooth enamel.

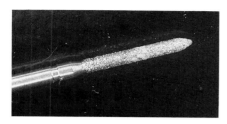

Fig. 4.36.
Diamond point bur.

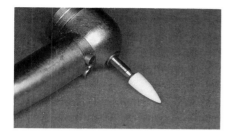

Fig. 4.37.
White stone bur.

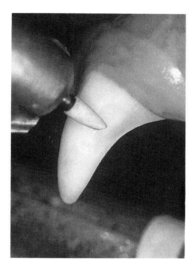

Fig. 4.38. White stone bur used to remove enamel defect.

Burs come in several shapes and sizes. The sizes are represented by numbers. The lower the number in a series, the smaller the bur head.

- **Round burs** are the most commonly used burs (Fig. 4.39). Their sizes range from 1/4 to 10. Round burs are used to create access holes when the pulp chamber is opened in preparation for endodontic treatment.

- **Pear-shaped burs**, sizes 330–333, are used to cut enamel and dentin for cavity preparation and to prepare undercuts for restoration retention.

- **Inverted cone burs** are shaped like an upside-down triangle (Fig. 4.40). Their sizes range from 33 1/2 to 37L (*L* indicates long). Inverted cones are used to prepare restoration sites for filling.

- **Fissure burs** have grooves on the head (Fig. 4.41). They are useful for sectioning teeth. Sides of the **straight fissure bur** are parallel. Sides of a **taper fissure bur** converge toward the tip. **Crosscut fissure burs** contain crosscuts along the blades, which act like the teeth of a saw to allow additional cutting. Common sizes for straight fissure burs range from 56 to 58L. Crosscut straight fissure burs range from 556 to 558L. Sizes for taper fissure burs range from 169 to 701L.

- **Trimming and finishing burs and disks** are designed for completing restorations (Fig. 4.42). The more blades there are, the finer the finish. For example, a 30-bladed bur, also known as a fine finishing bur, produces a smoother finish than does a 12-bladed bur. Finishing disks are available in various grades of abrasiveness, from coarse to very fine. They are used sequentially from coarse grade (to shape restorations) to fine grade (to smooth surfaces). The finest grade disk is used with a paste.

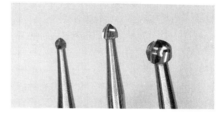

Fig. 4.39. Round burs sizes 2, 4, 8.

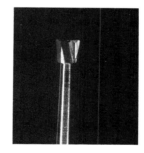

Fig. 4.40.
Inverted cone bur.

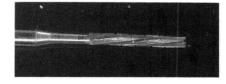

Fig. 4.41.
Fissure bur.

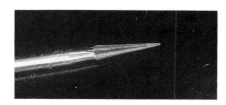

Fig. 4.42.
Finishing bur.

• **Cutting disks** are used to section teeth. Extreme caution must be taken to prevent harm to the patient or operator (Fig. 4.43).

After use, burs may be soaked briefly to prevent debris from drying. Do not soak carbides for longer than 20 minutes because chemicals in the soaking solutions may dull the burs. Debris may be removed from the burs with a nylon bristle brush or with the tip of a rubber eraser. Before the burs are placed in an autoclave, they are dipped in a corrosion inhibitor and placed on top of an autoclaveable bur block.

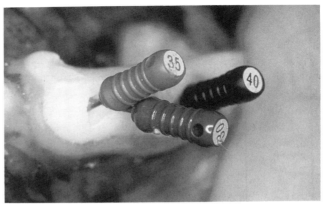

Fig. 4.44. Size 30, 35, and 40 files used during conventional root canal therapy in a maxillary fourth premolar.

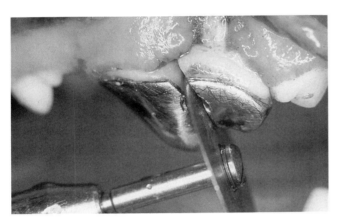

Fig. 4.43. Diamond disk used to section periodontally affected tooth.

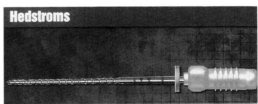

Fig. 4.45. Hedstrom (H) file. Courtesy of Tulsa Dental Products.

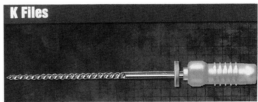

Fig. 4.46. K-files. Courtesy of Tulsa Dental Products.

ENDODONTIC INSTRUMENTS

The goal of endodontics is to seal the root apex to prevent infection and destruction of periapical support. Files, broaches, cements, fillers, and hand instruments are used to accomplish this goal.

Root canal files are hand instruments that come in gradually increasing sizes to enlarge, shape, and smooth the root canal (Fig. 4.44).

The most commonly used files in veterinary dentistry are the **Hedstrom (H)** (Fig. 4.45) and **Kerr (K)** files (Fig. 4.46). The lengths used depend on root canal length from tooth access to root apex. K files are available in lengths of 21 to 30 mm, while H files are as long as 60 mm. Most file widths are graded in ISO numbers from size 6 (0.6 mm at 1 mm from the tip) to size 140 (1.4 mm at 1 mm from the tip).

Tulsa Dental Products (Tulsa, Oklahoma) produces ProFile Series 29 files numbered from 1 to 11 (equivalent to ISO sizes 10–60) (Fig. 4.47). Successive Tulsa ProFile's files each increase in size by 29 percent. The consistent 29 percent graduated increase differs from the variation of ISO file widths, which vary between 8 and 50 percent between sizes. The ProFile 29 series files are more numerous in the smaller sizes.

Files are available with color-coded plastic handles that correlate with sizes 6–140 (0.6–1.4 mm at the tip). Manufacturers have agreed to make all number 10 file handles purple, the number 15 white, the number 20 yellow, and so on as noted in the following table. Most commonly used sizes for teeth other than large dog canines are the 8–45 widths at 21–25 mm lengths. Canine teeth of larger dogs require 50- to 60-mm files to reach the apex (Fig. 4.49). With repeated use, files will bend and eventually break. The safest practice is to use new files with each patient.

Endodontic stops are small round pieces of rubber or plastic that are placed on files to mark canal length (Fig. 4.50). An endodontic stop prevents the file from being placed through the root apex and harming the periapical tissues. The stop is placed on the file handle with the assistance of a radiograph to confirm the file is located at the apex (the distance from the tooth's access to the apex is the file's **working length**).

> ❧ **FILE HANDLE COLORS**

Purple	size 10
White	size 15
Yellow	size 20
Red	size 25
Blue	size 30
Green	size 35
Black	size 40

Gates Glidden drills are small flame-shaped rotary cutting instruments with long shanks (Fig. 4.51). They are used with slow speed contra-angle handpieces to enlarge the root canal in order to allow easy access for filing. They are sized from 1 to 6 based on the blade's width (6 is the widest).

Barbed broaches are short handled instruments used to withdraw pulp, absorbent points, and other debris from the root canal (Fig. 4.52). They are available in 25-, 30-, 45-, and 50-mm lengths and 15- to 40-mm widths.

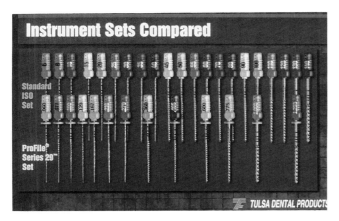

Fig. 4.47. Comparison of ISO file sizes with ProFile series 29 sizes. Courtesy of Tulsa Dental Products.

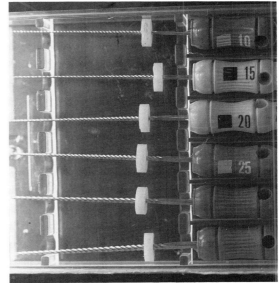

Fig. 4.50. Endodontic files with stops attached.

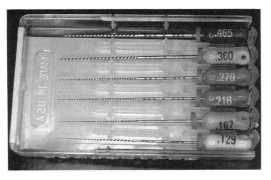

Fig. 4.48. Package of endodontic files (Tulsa Dental Products).

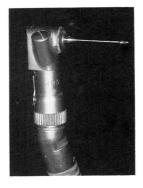

Fig. 4.51. Gates Glidden Drill attached to 10:1 reduction gear on low-speed drill.

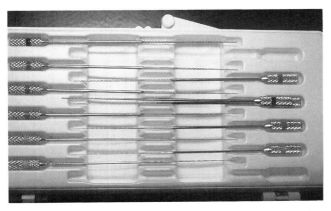

Fig. 4.49. Sixty-mm Hedstrom endodontic files (Henry Schein, Inc.).

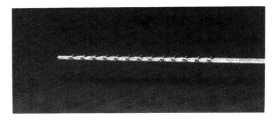

Fig. 4.52. Barbed broach.

Spiral paste fillers, also called Lentulo spirals, come in 25-, 30-, and 45- to 60-mm lengths (Fig. 4.53). They are used to carry root canal sealer into the prepared root canal before placement of gutta-percha. They may be used by hand or at very low speeds in a latch-type contra-angle handpiece with a 10:1 reduction gear.

Retrograde amalgam fillers are used to apply calcium hydroxide or amalgam for vital pulpotomies and apical sealer in surgical endodontics (Figs. 4.54 and 4.55).

College tipped pliers, also called cotton pliers, enable the operator to pick up and hold paper points or gutta-percha points in place to insert into the prepared root canal (Fig. 4.56). Pliers are also used to hold cotton pledgets to clean tooth surfaces. They are available in both locking and nonlocking styles, as well as with plain or serrated tips.

Spatulas are instruments used to mix dental materials. Wide, broad, flexible spatulas are used to mix impression materials, plaster, and stone. Cement spatulas are thinner and nonflexible. Special Teflon spatulas may be used when mixing and delivering composite material to avoid discoloration during the mixing process.

Pluggers, also called condensers, have straight tips with flat ends (Fig. 4.57). They are used to compress

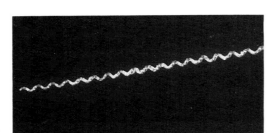

Fig. 4.53. Spiral paste filler.

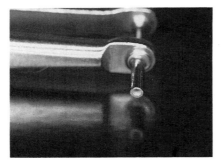

Fig. 4.54. Retrograde amalgam filler.

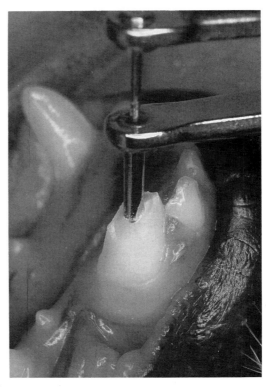

Fig. 4.55. Retrograde amalgam filler used to apply calcium hydoxide in crown reduction procedure.

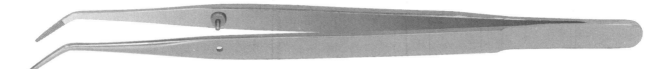

Fig. 4.56. College tipped pliers.

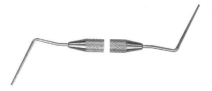

Fig. 4.57. Endodontic pluggers.

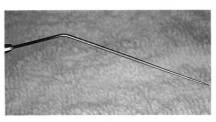

Fig. 4.58. Holmstrom spreader (Cislak Manufacturing, Inc.).

gutta-percha vertically toward the root apex. Pluggers are either handheld or finger gripped. They also come in numerous sizes and lengths.

Spreaders are used to condense gutta-percha laterally and apically in the prepared canal. Holmstrom spreaders/pluggers (Cislak Manufacturing, Inc.) are of sufficient size to reach the apex of most canine teeth (Fig. 4.58). When heated, the spreader is used to melt and pack gutta-percha into the canal space (Fig. 4.59).

Paper points, also referred to as absorbent points, are sterile, absorbent, narrow, rolled papers. Paper points are used to dry the cleaned canal before filling. Paper points come in assorted widths (from xx-fine to coarse) and lengths to adapt to the canal being treated. They are often handled with locking college tipped pliers.

Curing lights are used in the restoration process to promote polymerization in glass ionomer cements and/or composite resins (Fig. 4.60). Curing lights come as handheld gun types or wands connected with a fiber-optic cable to the console. Handheld curing lights resist wear and tear better than the wand type, and usually only the bulb needs replacement, not the expensive fiber-optic cord.

HAND INSTRUMENTS

Understanding the purpose and use of hand instruments is basic to veterinary dental practice (Fig. 4.62). Clinical results obtained for the patient depend in part on the proficiency with which instruments are used. The main purpose of using hand instruments is to create an environment in which tissues can heal and their health be maintained.

Each instrument is designed for a specific application during calculus removal and root planing. A clear understanding of the relationship of the cutting edge or edges to the other parts of the instrument is essential for correct angulation during instrumentation and for positioning on the sharpening stone.

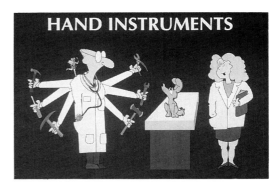

Fig. 4.61.

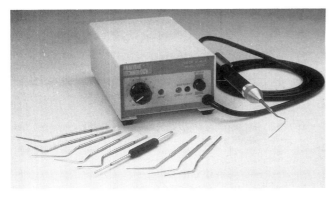

Fig. 4.59. Touch 'n Heat thermal spreader and plugger (CK Dental Specialties).

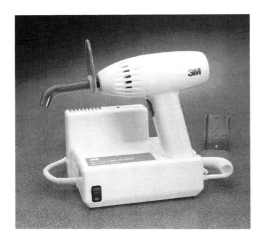

Fig. 4.60. Curing light.

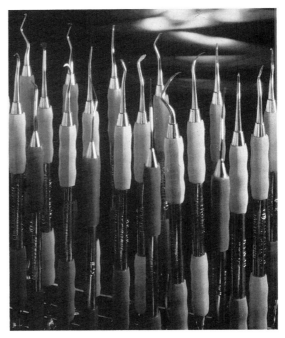

Fig. 4.62. Hand instruments.

Anatomy of the Hand Instrument

The hand instrument (Fig. 4.63) has

- A **handle** for grasping, which may be solid or hollow

- A **shank**, which connects the handle to the working end and allows adaptation of the working end to tooth surfaces

- A **working end**, which does the work of the instrument. Hand instruments have either one or two working ends. The working end is made up of a face, cutting edge, back, and toe.

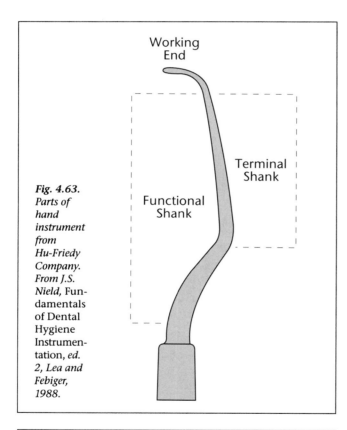

Working End

Terminal Shank

Functional Shank

Fig. 4.63. Parts of hand instrument from Hu-Friedy Company. From J.S. Nield, Fundamentals of Dental Hygiene Instrumentation, *ed. 2, Lea and Febiger, 1988.*

> ✧ **HAND INSTRUMENTS USED TO DIAGNOSE AND TREAT PERIODONTAL DISEASE**
> - The sickle-shaped supragingival scaler
> - The subgingival curette
> - The Shepherd's hook explorer
> - The graduated periodontal probe.
>   One- to 3-mm graduations are marked as indented lines or painted blocks.
> - The periosteal elevator

Hand Instrument Identification

- The **classification** of the hand instrument is determined by its use. Examples of classification include periodontal probes, explorers, curettes, sickles, and chisels.

  — Periodontal probes and explorers are detection instruments. The probe is used for measuring the depth of periodontal pockets. The explorer is used to detect calculus, irregularities in the tooth surface, and pulpal exposure.
  — Curettes are used for gross scaling to remove large calculus deposits, definitive scaling to remove fine calculus, and root planing to smooth and polish the cemental surfaces.
  — Sickles and chisels are also used in gross calculus removal but are not suitable for definitive scaling or root planing.

- The **instrument design/number** bears the name of the school or individual responsible for the instrument's development. A number provides more specific identification of a design. A double-ended instrument may have a pair of numbers that identify working ends. Gracey curettes, for example, are produced by several manufacturers. Gracey is the name of the individual who designed a particular series of curettes, which are numbered from 1 to 14. Although the superficial appearance of the instruments may be similar, close examination of the handle, shank, and working end of each will reveal differences that can be significant when you use the instrument.

Hand Positioning

Hand instruments are generally held in a **modified pen grasp** (Fig. 4.64). This provides maximum control of the instrument and a wide range of movement. The instrument is held between tips of the thumb and index finger, near the junction between the handle and shank. The handle rests against the hand between the thumb and knuckles.

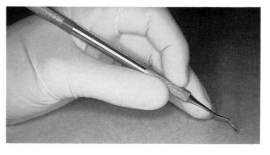

Fig. 4.64. Modified pen grasp.

The middle finger is used to guide the instrument and to detect rough surfaces. The index and middle fingers are bent. Fingers must be relaxed while holding a hand instrument. The little finger (pinkie) has no function in this grasp and should be held close to the ring finger in a relaxed, comfortable manner.

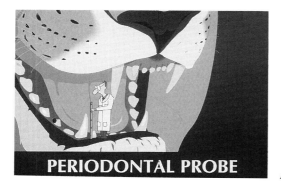

Fig. 4.65.

The Periodontal Probe

A periodontal probe is used to measure sulcus and pocket depths. This thin, dipsticklike device is marked in 1- to 3-mm increments. As the instrument is inserted into the gingival sulcus, depths can be read and recorded. The procedure of taking millimeter readings is known as probing. Circumferential probing is done at four points on a tooth. Normal sulcus depth in the dog is 2 mm or less; in the cat, 1 mm or less. Greater depths may indicate periodontal disease and require treatment.

Radiographs indicate areas of bone loss where pockets may occur, but they cannot be used to detect or measure periodontal pockets because pockets represent soft tissue changes. Using the probe also gives the practitioner invaluable information concerning gingival bleeding, an important sign of inflammation, and the depth, shape, and tissue characteristics of the pocket.

Probes vary in cross-sectional design and millimeter markings (Fig. 4.66). They may be rectangular (flat), oval, or round. The calibrated working end is marked in millimeters at varying intervals to facilitate reading of depth measurements. Readings greater than 5 mm are important to note because most pockets deeper than 5

mm will need surgical care (a flap procedure or extraction).

The **Marquis probe** is color coded by alternately colored bands that mark 3, 6, 9, and 12 mm (Fig. 4.67). This probe has a thin working end. Care must be taken in estimating the millimeter readings between the markings.

The **Williams probe** is marked at 1, 2, 3 and then 5, 7, 8, 9, and 10 mm. Be careful when purchasing a Williams probe because some manufacturers produce a working end that is too thick to allow easy insertion.

The **Michigan-O** probe is marked at 3, 6, and 8 mm. Many veterinarians prefer this probe because it has a very thin working end. The Michigan-O probe can be obtained with Williams markings.

Periodontal measurements are taken by inserting the probe under the free gingival margin and gently moving it to the bottom of the sulcus or pocket. Keep the probe parallel to the tooth surface to ensure correct measurement. After inserting, gently "walk" the tip along the bottom of the pocket. This walking technique allows an accurate measurement of the level of attachment around the tooth. The measurements are recorded for multiple points on each tooth.

Probing depths are measured from the base of the pocket to the margin of the free gingiva. Normal depths for dogs are 2 mm or less; for cats, 1 mm or less.

The level of attachment (loss of attachment) is measured from the cemento-enamel junction (CEJ) to the apical extent of the sulcus or pocket. When the gingival margin coincides with the CEJ, the level of attachment and the pocket depth are equal; when the gingival margin is located apical to the CEJ, the loss of attachment is greater than the pocket depth. *The level of attachment of the epithelium at the base of the pocket is of greater diagnostic significance than the probing depth of the pocket.*

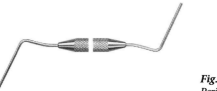

Fig. 4.66.
Periodontal probes.

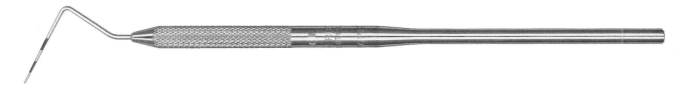

Fig. 4.67. Marquis periodontal probe.

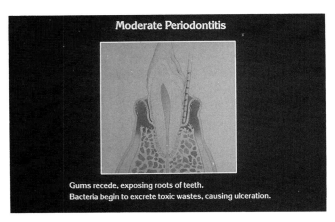

Moderate Periodontitis

Gums recede, exposing roots of teeth.
Bacteria begin to excrete toxic wastes, causing ulceration.

Fig. 4.68.

How does determining the level of attachment help the veterinarian? The probe provides an "under-the-gum-line" look at dental pathology and is an essential part of every dental examination. If there are areas of abnormal depth, radiographs are taken, and the client is advised of a therapy plan (flap surgery, bone graft, hemisection and endodontics, or extraction).

The Dental Explorer

The dental explorer has a sharp point used to discover dental defects (Fig. 4.69). Explorers are helpful for examining the root surface for calculus, resorptive lesions, necrotic cementum, and areas of pulpal exposure. An explorer is the most sensitive instrument for tactile conduction. Never use an explorer to remove calculus. The working end of the explorer is 1–2 mm in length and is called the tip. The entire tip should be adapted to the tooth during instrumentation.

Interpretation of subgingival conditions with the dental explorer:

- **Normal**—Your fingers on the instrument handle will not feel any interruptions in the path of the explorer when it is inserted and withdrawn from the sulcus or pocket.

- **Ledge of subgingival calculus present**—The explorer moves over the tooth surface, encounters a ledge, moves laterally over it, and returns to the tooth surface.

- **Fine deposits of subgingival calculus**—Instead of a definite interruption, there is a gritty sensation as the explorer passes over fine calculus.

- **Carious lesion**—Proceeding along the tooth surface to the base of the pocket, the explorer dips in and then comes out again.

The Scaler

The scaler is designed to remove dental deposits from tooth surfaces above the gum line and to smooth the tooth so it will resist reaccumulation of these deposits (Fig. 4.70). The scaler's blade is triangular, with two cutting edges that converge to form a point. The blade design prohibits subgingival insertion because it may injure the sulcus. *Do not try to use the scaler subgingivally*.

A scaler is used supragingivally with the blade apical to the deposit and the side of the tip contacting the tooth surface. A short, coronal pull stroke directed in line with the long axis of the tooth is used to remove supragingival debris.

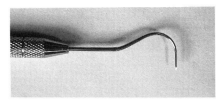

Fig. 4.69. Dental explorer (Cbi).

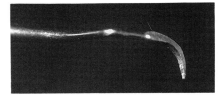

Fig. 4.70. Dental scaler.

The Curette

Curettes are similar to scalers but have a smooth, rounded heel opposite the cutting surface. A rounded back makes curettes less traumatic to soft tissues. Curettes are used to remove subgingival calculus, for root planing, and for curettage (removal of disease in the soft tissue of the periodontal pocket). Periodontal debridement's goal is to restore gingival health by removal of tooth and root surface irritants. Bacterial plaque and debris are toxic to the tooth's support structures. Removal of calculus is necessary because calculus acts as a retention site for bacteria and toxins, eventually causing and supporting periodontal disease.

Universal curettes have one blade with two cutting edges and a rounded toe for use on mesial and distal surfaces. Both cutting edges may be used on the front and back of a tooth. The nearest working end should be parallel to the long axis of the tooth. Popular universal curettes include Columbia, McCall, Barnhart, and Langer styles.

Area-specific curettes are designed to adapt to a specific area or tooth surface. To tell if a curette is universal or area specific, hold the instrument with the working end toward you and the terminal shank perpendicular to the ground. If the working end's face is 90 degrees to the ground, it is a universal curette. Area-specific curettes are offset at 70 degrees. The lower cutting edge is the one to use next to the tooth surface. The Gracey is an example of an area-specific curette.

- Commonly used area-specific curettes are the **Gracey curette** 11/12 and 13/14. The Gracey has only one cutting edge, which is designed for removal of deep subgingival calculus, for root planing, and for curettage of the periodontal pocket (Fig. 4.71).

- **Langer curettes** are designed with the shank of a Gracey combined with a universal blade design. These instruments can scale both mesial and distal surfaces.

- The **after-five series** is made up of Gracey curettes designed with a terminal shank that is 3 mm longer than that of standard Gracey curettes. This allows improved access to deep periodontal pockets and root surfaces. After-fives feature a thin blade to ease gingival insertion and reduce tissue distention.

- Other curettes are depicted in Figures 4.72–4.74.

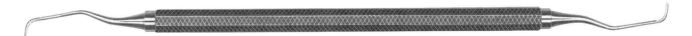

Fig. 4.71. *Gracey curette.*

Basic Prophylaxis Setup*
Complete set-up designed to handle routine diagnostic and prophy procedures.

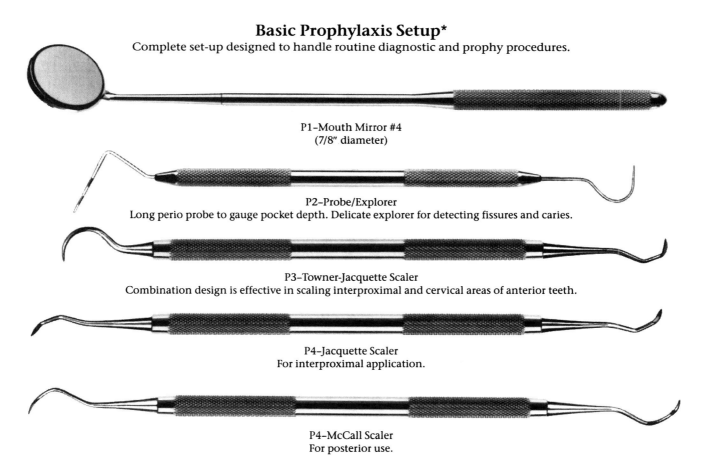

P1–Mouth Mirror #4
(7/8" diameter)

P2–Probe/Explorer
Long perio probe to gauge pocket depth. Delicate explorer for detecting fissures and caries.

P3–Towner-Jacquette Scaler
Combination design is effective in scaling interproximal and cervical areas of anterior teeth.

P4–Jacquette Scaler
For interproximal application.

P4–McCall Scaler
For posterior use.

Fig. 4.72. *Basic dental hand instruments. Courtesy of Cislak Manufacturing, Inc.*

Additional Prophylaxis Instruments

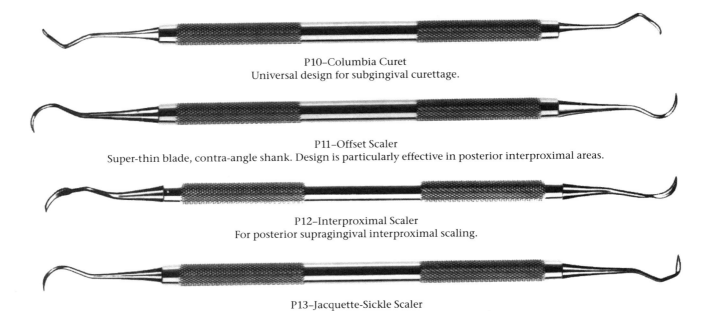

P10–Columbia Curet
Universal design for subgingival curettage.

P11–Offset Scaler
Super-thin blade, contra-angle shank. Design is particularly effective in posterior interproximal areas.

P12–Interproximal Scaler
For posterior supragingival interproximal scaling.

P13–Jacquette-Sickle Scaler
A more delicate design than our P3 Towner/Jacquette scaler.

Periodontal Subgingival Scalers
Area-specific curets designed with rigid shanks for greater strength.

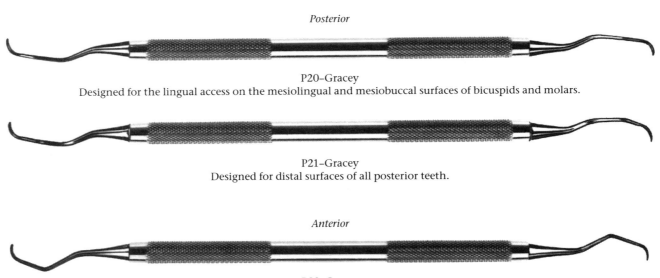

Posterior

P20–Gracey
Designed for the lingual access on the mesiolingual and mesiobuccal surfaces of bicuspids and molars.

P21–Gracey
Designed for distal surfaces of all posterior teeth.

Anterior

P22–Gracey
Short contra-angle, for adaptability on incisors and cuspids.

Fig. 4.73. *Additional hand instruments. Courtesy of Cislak Manufacturing, Inc.*

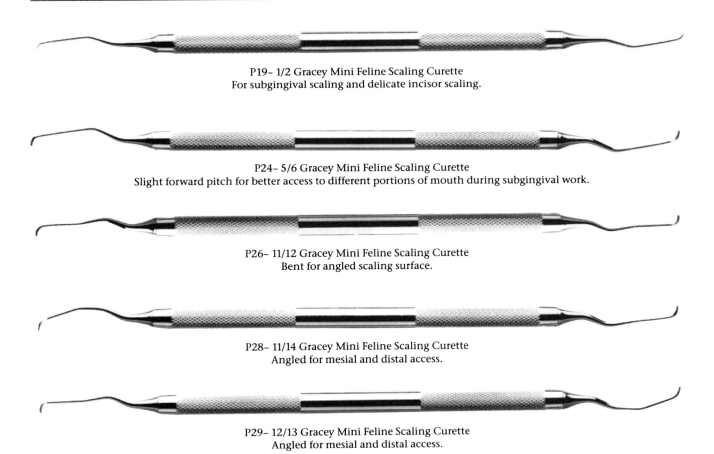

P19– 1/2 Gracey Mini Feline Scaling Curette
For subgingival scaling and delicate incisor scaling.

P24– 5/6 Gracey Mini Feline Scaling Curette
Slight forward pitch for better access to different portions of mouth during subgingival work.

P26– 11/12 Gracey Mini Feline Scaling Curette
Bent for angled scaling surface.

P28– 11/14 Gracey Mini Feline Scaling Curette
Angled for mesial and distal access.

P29– 12/13 Gracey Mini Feline Scaling Curette
Angled for mesial and distal access.

Fig. 4.74. *Feline scalers and curettes. Courtesy of Cislak Manufacturing, Inc.*

It is important to adapt the working end of the hand instrument to the tooth surface. The portion of the cutting edge in contact with the tooth will vary, depending on the tooth surface involved.

The best way to use a curette is to maintain the terminal shank parallel to the tooth surface. This will aid in engaging the working blade's cutting edge. Focus on using the distal third of the instrument toe on the tooth surface. The instrument is inserted into the sulcus with the blade face parallel to the root surface until it engages the bottom. Then the curette is rotated until the terminal shank is parallel to the root surface. This step usually engages calculus and/or debris subgingivally. The instrument is then pulled coronally, with the engaged material drawn toward the cemento-enamel junction. The process is repeated in circumferentially overlapping strokes until the root surface is smooth.

Periodontal Surgery Instruments

Periodontal surgery instruments include the Molt elevator (Fig. 4.75), Freer elevator (Fig. 4.76), Ochsenbein chisels (Fig. 4.77), and Cislak Manufacturing thin periodontal surgical instruments (Fig. 4.78).

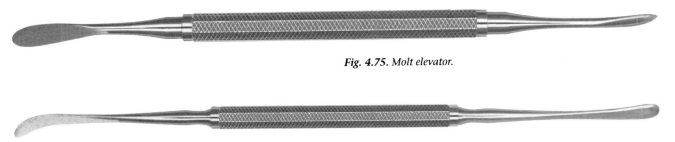

Fig. 4.75. *Molt elevator.*

Fig. 4.76. *Freer elevator.*

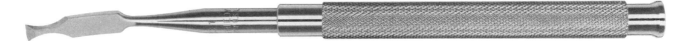

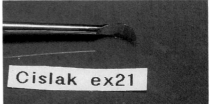

Fig. 4.77. Ochsenbein chisel.

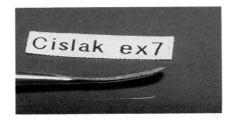

Fig. 4.78. Thin periodontal surgical instruments especially suited for canine and feline flap surgery (Cislak Manufacturing, Inc.).

Extraction Hand Instruments

Elevators are placed between the tooth's root and alveolar bone to exert pressure on the periodontal ligament so that the tooth may be extracted. The basic components of an elevator are the handle, shank, and blade or tip. Some elevators also have serrated ridges on the cutting edge to sever the periodontal ligament.

Care is essential when using elevators. The operator must be sure the root has a clear unobstructed path of exit. *The use of force to bypass an obstruction of bone will either fracture the bone, tooth, or both.* Lever action is used for prying a tooth root tip from its socket. The elevator engages the tooth through a purchase point (a groove or hole in the tooth that is made with a bur) or through

the operator gripping the tooth with the edge of the blade and using bone as a fulcrum to lift the tooth out of its socket. Torquing the handle and holding it for at least 30 seconds will help fatigue the periodontal ligament, causing bleeding that will help push out the tooth.

The number 301 (Fig. 4.79), 302, and 303 elevators are commonly used in small animal dental practice. Their thin tips are especially suited for teasing out small roots. The number 34-S and number 46 elevators have thicker tips and may cause damage if excess force is applied.

Luxators are elevators with wide, thin tips. They are designed for comfort and control during tooth extractions and are especially suited for small animal extrac-

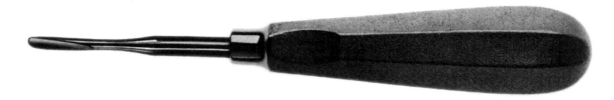

Fig. 4.79. Number 301 elevator. Courtesy of Cislak Manufacturing, Inc.

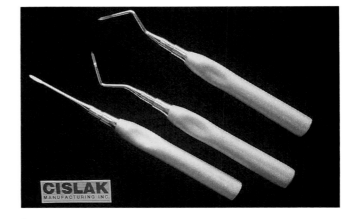

Fig. 4.80. Root tip picks.

tions. The blade's tip is thin and can be easily inserted in the sulcular space to sever the periodontal ligament. Some helpful hints for use of luxators:

- Place the luxator tip in the periodontal space on the mesial side of the root. Using moderate pressure, insert the luxator to two-thirds the length of the root and apply axial rotation (5–10 degrees). The thumb and index finger will immediately feel any dislocation of the luxator. Do not use the luxator as a lever.

- If the root remains firm, the same procedure is repeated on the distal side. Contact with the root surface is maintained at all times. After mesial and distal luxation, the tooth should be dislodged.

- Gentle torque pressure is placed on the tooth to be extracted. Eventually (within minutes), the tooth will loosen and become mobile.

- The maxillary lateral incisors must be dislodged in a palatal direction because of their root angles.

Extraction forceps are used for removing loosened teeth from the alveolar bone (Fig. 4.81). The forceps are composed of three parts: a handle, hinge, and beak. The handle allows the instrument to be grasped to deliver adequate leverage and pressure to the beak. Care must be taken not to apply excessive pressure or torque to extraction forceps because it may fracture the tooth or alveolar bone.

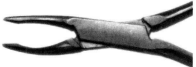

Fig. 4.81. Extraction forceps. Courtesy of Cislak Manufacturing, Inc.

EX31
Friedman Rongeur Delicate
(14 cm/5 ¹/₂″)

Hand Instrument Sharpening

Why hand instruments should be sharpened:

- To improve calculus removal
- To save time
- To improve tactile sensitivity
- To minimize animal discomfort
- To reduce hand fatigue
- To reduce risk of trauma to soft tissues

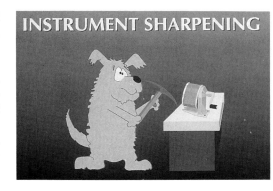

Fig. 4.82.

How to recognize a dull instrument:

- The instrument does not "grab" or "bite."
- More pressure is necessary for effective instrumentation.
- The dental procedure takes longer than usual.

How to determine instrument sharpness:

- **Plastic stick test**—Apply the cutting edge to a conical plastic stick to evaluate the bite as the edge takes hold. If there is no bite, the instrument needs sharpening.

- **Visual inspection**—A bright light and magnifying glass are used to inspect the instrument. Rotate the blade until the edge is facing the light. If you can see light reflecting off the cutting edge, then the instrument is dull.

Before each use, scalers and curettes must be sharpened and then sterilized. A dull, rounded surface cuts only with excessive force, if it cuts at all. The goal of instrument sharpening is to convert a flattened, dull surface into a sharp cutting edge while preserving the original blade shape.

Sharpening is performed to retain the 70- to 80-degree angle between the face and lateral-working surface of a scaler or curette. The flat **Arkansas sharpening stone** is a general-purpose natural stone that may be adapted for use on most instruments. The Arkansas stone has fine grit. Oil lubrication is suggested when using this stone; however, it can be used dry. The oil serves as a vehicle to float metal particles as they are ground from the blade, and it prevents those shavings from becoming imbedded in the stone.

The **India stone** can be used for sharpening excessively dull instruments (Fig. 4.83). The India stone is man-made, composed of aluminum oxide crystals with fine or medium grit. Oil lubrication is required when sharpening with this stone.

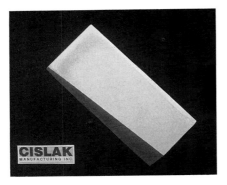

Fig. 4.83. India sharpening stone. Courtesy of Cislak Manufacturing, Inc.

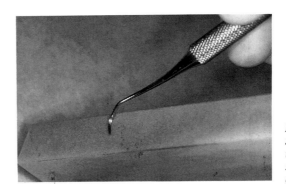

Fig. 4.84. Sharpening an instrument on a stone.

The **ceramic stone** is a hard synthetic stone available in either fine or medium grit. This stone is excellent for routine sharpening of dental instruments and uses water for lubrication.

Stone shapes:

• **Conical**—The conical stone is an Arkansas stone used for finishing or removing any wire edges after sharpening.
• **Flat**—The flat stone typically is rectangular but comes in various sizes. It can be an Arkansas, ceramic, or India stone.
• **Wedge**—The wedge stone is a rectangular-shaped stone with rounded edges and commonly is an Arkansas or India stone.

Care of sharpening stones:

• After repeated use, stones may become blackened. They are maintained using ammonia, gasoline, or kerosene.

• Stones should be stored in a covered container with a light coat of oil to prevent drying.

• If the stone has become glazed from repeated use and has lost its abrasive qualities, rub it over fine emery paper for resurfacing.

• Autoclaving can be used to sterilize the stone.

• Use a sterile stone when sharpening sterile instruments.

To sharpen, an instrument can be moved across a stationary stone (Fig. 4.84), or the instrument can be held stationary and the stone moved.

STEPS FOR INSTRUMENT SHARPENING–STATIONARY STONE TECHNIQUE

Using a gauze sponge, lubricate an Arkansas or India stone with a thin layer of light machine oil. Ceramic stones should be lubricated with a few drops of water.

1. Place the stone on a flat surface.
2. While holding the instrument at the correct angle against the stone, pull the instrument in 1-in. strokes several times.
3. Wipe instruments and check for sharpness.

STATIONARY INSTRUMENT–MOVING STONE TECHNIQUE

1. Place the stone in your dominant hand.
2. Stabilize the instrument on the edge of a countertop with the palm of the nondominant hand.
3. Point the toe of the instrument toward you with the face parallel to the floor.
4. Place the stone against the instrument at the instrument's heel, establishing a 110-degree angle between the cutting edge and the stone.
5. Start sharpening in short up and down strokes and finish with a down stroke.
6. For universal curettes repeat the procedure to sharpen the opposite cutting edge.
7. Wipe the instrument and check for sharpness.

STEPS FOR INSTRUMENT SHARPENING USING A CONICAL STONE

1. Stabilize instrument.
2. Place stone at junction of face and shank.
3. Role stone across the face, moving toward the toe.

EQUIPMENT MAINTENANCE

Dental handpieces are precision pieces of equipment. They must be maintained to ensure proper operation and maximum life. All handpieces require daily lubrication.

- At the end of *each day,* scrub the handpiece with a cleaning solution to remove soil and debris. A gauze, sponge, or brush may be used.

- Then rinse the handpiece without immersion.

- Thoroughly dry the handpiece using gauze, paper towels, or air from the air/water syringe.

- According to manufacturer instructions, add lubricant to the middle-sized hole at the connection area (Fig. 4.85).

- Briefly run the handpiece to remove excess lubricant.

Cleaning and lubricating the right-angle handpiece:

- Place the working end of the handpiece into a small bottle of handpiece cleaning solvent.

- Run the handpiece backward and forward for one minute in each direction.

- Remove the handpiece from the cleaner and wipe it dry.

- Disassemble the handpiece using the special wrench furnished by the manufacturer.

- Place heavy lubricant (petroleum jelly) on the gears of the handpiece before it is reassembled.

Maintenance of high-speed delivery systems:

- **Air storage tank**—Condensation will build up in the air storage tank. Depending on the humidity in your environment, condensation should be drained weekly to monthly (Fig. 4.86).

- **Compressor**—Unless you have an oil-free compressor, an oil level indicator or dipstick is attached to the compressor tank (Fig. 4.87). The level and color must be checked monthly.

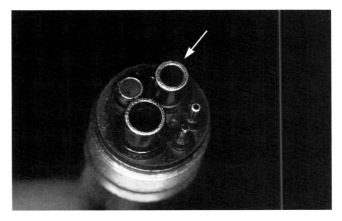

Fig. 4.85. Oil is applied to the next to largest opening for maintenance of the high-speed handpiece (arrow).

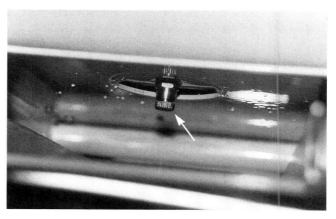

Fig. 4.86. Pressure tank drain.

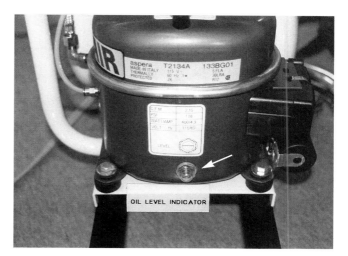

Fig. 4.87. Oil level indicator (arrow).

> **PREVENTIVE COMPRESSOR MAINTENANCE**

	WEEKLY	MONTLY	ANNUALLY
Check oil level. Correct level is between maximum and minimum indications while at a standstill. Do not overfill.		•	
Drain tank (at a maximum pressure of 30 psi).	•		
Check compressor and air line for leaks.		•	
Give compressor overall visual check and wipe with soft rag. If necessary, use paraffin on rag to remove sticky adhesions. Dust and dirt prevent cooling.		•	
Clean or replace intake filter.			•
Operate safety valve by gently pulling protruding rod.			•

Infection Control

Sometimes, dental procedures involve infected tissues in patients that may have compromised immune systems. Operation of high-speed delivery systems generates bacteria-laden aerosols, which contaminate the operatory room, so these must be used in an area away from open surgical sites.

- Those performing dental therapy must wear face masks to help prevent inhalation of pathogens.

- Protective eyewear is also required to guard against debris and aerosol injuring the operator's eyes.

- Before periodontal therapy, patient treatment with antibiotics for periodontal pathogens decreases bacteremia and aerosol contamination.

- Disinfection of the oral cavity by rinsing with a 0.2 percent chlorhexidine solution before periodontal therapy will also reduce the number of bacteria.

- Use a new pair of exam gloves for each patient. Dental procedures must be performed under general anesthesia with a cuffed endotracheal tube in place and the pharynx packed with absorbent material.

- The patient's head should be angled downward to promote drainage.

Precautions must be observed to prevent patient cross infection:

- New gloves should be worn for each patient.

- A sterilized set of instruments should be used for each animal. Instrument cassettes are autoclaveable.

- For each patient, individual containers of prophy paste are used, or a new tongue depressor is used to scoop out the prophy paste from a larger receptacle before use.

Feline patients require special concern because feline leukemia and feline immunodeficiency viruses may be transmitted by blood or saliva. Virus particles can be passed between patients through dental procedures. A virus may become lodged in prophy paste remaining on the head of the prophy angle and then transmitted to the next patient even if the prophy cup is changed. Because of this, *disposable prophy head use is mandatory for feline patients.*

Sterilization

Dental instruments used in the mouth must be sterile. Sterilization kills all microorganisms. The sterilization procedure is straightforward:

- All instruments need to be cleaned before they are sterilized.

- They are first washed with a noncorrosive detergent.

- After dental instruments are cleaned, they are bagged or wrapped before sterilization.

- The autoclave is a steam chamber where instruments to be sterilized are placed. During the sterilization cycle, distilled water flows into the chamber and is heated to create steam. Since the chamber is sealed, pressure increases to approximately 15 psi. This increase in pressure causes the heat to rise to approximately 250°F. When instruments are exposed to this high pressure/high temperature steam for 15 minutes, sterilization occurs.

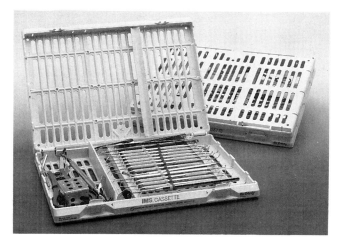

Fig. 4.88. Instrument cassette. Courtesy of Hu-Friedy Company.

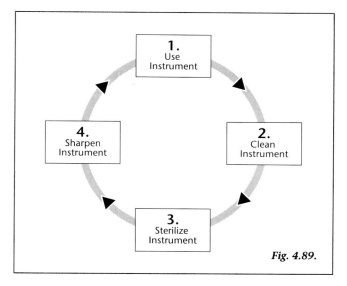

1.
Use
Instrument

2.
Clean
Instrument

3.
Sterilize
Instrument

4.
Sharpen
Instrument

Fig. 4.89.

Disinfection

Disinfection is the process of destroying microbial life. Chemical disinfection will not eliminate all viruses and spores. The term "cold sterilization" has been applied to the process of immersing instruments into chemicals at room temperature. This is a misnomer, since only disinfection, not sterilization, occurs. Heat and pressure are superior for killing pathogens.

DENTAL MATERIALS

Teeth-Cleaning, Periodontal, and Hygiene Products

Prophy paste or flour pumice is used to polish teeth once the supra- and subgingival calculus is removed. Polishing must be performed after every professional teeth cleaning to remove microscratches caused by the cleaning. Polishing teeth decreases surface area of enamel, which retards plaque recolonization. Polishing also removes microplaque.

Silicone dioxide paste and zirconium silicate paste are most commonly used for polishing.

Prophy paste or flour pumice is applied with a prophy cup attached to the prophy angle on a low-speed handpiece. The paste is taken from its container with a tongue depressor and applied either to the prophy cup or to the teeth. Prophy angles have screw-on or snap-on fittings. Polishing involves a light touch for only seconds per tooth. The prophy cup's edge should flare under the gingival margin. A final rinse to remove remaining paste and debris is necessary.

Disclosing agents are organic dyes that reveal areas of dental plaque (Fig. 4.90). They are useful both in diagnosis and in assessing the efficiency of cleansing procedures. A disclosing agent is swabbed on tooth surfaces using cotton pledgets. Excess solution is rinsed off with water. Caution must be used when applying the solution to the teeth of light-haired breeds. The solution may temporarily stain facial hairs, which could upset your client.

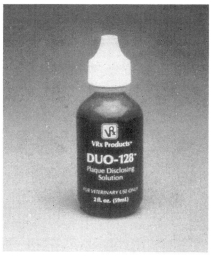

Fig. 4.90. Disclosing agent (VRX Pharmaceuticals).

Fluoride use has many advantages in veterinary dentistry.

- It enters enamel and creates fluorapatite, which strengthens the tooth.

- It reduces tooth sensitivity from exposed dentinal tubules.

- Stannous fluoride destroys certain bacteria-decreasing plaque.

Fluoride, applied topically, is supplied as a varnish, mouthwash, foam, spray, solution, or gel incorporated in toothpaste.

- **Varnish** and **mouthwash** fluoride products are rarely used on small animals.

- **Foam** fluoride is supplied as Flurafom (VRX Pharmaceuticals, Harbor City, California). Sodium fluoride (2 percent) is applied after teeth cleaning. The foam is allowed to dry in the mouth without irrigation for at least three minutes before the anesthetized animal awakes.

- A 0.02 percent sodium fluoride CET Oral Hygiene **Spray** (VRX Pharmaceuticals) is available for home care.

- Stannous fluoride is available as an 8 percent topically applied **solution** or in a home care Qygel 0.4 percent **gel** (Veterinary Product Labs, Phoenix, Arizona).

- Sodium monofluorophosphate fluoride is popularly used in veterinary dentistry as part of CET **Toothpaste** (VRX Pharmaceuticals).

Chlorhexidine solution (0.1-0.2 percent) is used in veterinary medicine as an adjunct to periodontal therapy. *Chlorhexidine is the most effective chemical agent available for the prevention and reduction of plaque accumulation and gingivitis.*
Positive properties of chlorhexidine include

- Being an effective antiseptic with broad-spectrum antimicrobial activity

- Inhibiting plaque development by binding to the pellicle, which reduces absorption of plaque by the tooth surface

- Rendering existing plaque nonpathogenic, which prevents production of the plaque's harmful by-products

- Promoting resolution of accompanying gingivitis when chlorhexidine is used after periodontal surgery for one to two weeks

- Aiding wound healing after oral surgery by preventing or resolving secondary bacterial infection

- When used before ultrasonic scaling, decreasing both the operator's exposure to aerosolized bacteria and the patient's to bacteremia

There are some minor disadvantages to the use of chlorhexidine in animals:

- It has a bitter taste, especially to cats.

- It stains teeth brown or black, but this is easily removed at prophy time.

The gluconate form of chlorhexidine is most commonly used as an irrigating solution, a daily oral rinse, or a part of the 0.12 percent toothbrushing dentifrice CHX Gel (VRX Pharmaceuticals) or Dentivet Toothpaste (Virbac, Fort Worth, Texas).

The aqueous preparation diffuses more easily to a wide area of the mouth than the gel does. Unfortunately, to be effective, chlorhexidine must stay in contact with the affected tissues for at least two minutes. For this reason the gel is preferred.

The acetate form of chlorhexidine is available as Oral Fresh (Cislak Manufacturing, Inc., Burbank, Illinois) and may not be as soluble as the gluconate form. Initial use of the solution or gel should be twice daily for two weeks, followed by daily application.

Zinc ascorbate is available for veterinary use as Maxiguard oral cleansing gel (Addison Biological Laboratory, Inc., Fayette, Missouri). This product is used to promote healing after periodontal surgery and to reduce halitosis.

Lactoperoxidase and **glucose oxidase** stimulate the salivary peroxidase system to help control plaque. They are available in CET Enzymatic Dentifrice (VRX Pharmaceuticals).

Endodontic Materials

Zinc phosphate cement is often used on top of gutta-percha and below composite cement. Its high compressive strength and thermal insulating properties make it a useful cement on vital teeth.

Gutta-percha is a combination of zinc oxide eugenol, rubber, and barium. It is used as core-filling material in endodontics. Gutta-percha has properties of being radiodense, bacteriostatic, nonirritating, and able to be condensed laterally and apically. Gutta-percha points are slender, tapered, and pointed to fit contours of the root canal. As with the paper points, various widths and lengths are available. During root canal therapy, multiple points are condensed into the canal space until it is completely filled.

Heat will soften gutta-percha. Softened material fills the canal space more easily than hard cones do. Heat can be applied via Bunsen burner flames to endodontic spreaders, or special instruments (Touch 'n Heat, CK Dental Specialties, Orange, California) are used to apply heat to gutta-percha. Chloroform will also soften gutta-percha and can be used in a "chloropercha technique" to make gutta-percha easier to work with.

Zinc oxide-eugenol (ZOE) is a cement used to seal the root apex and to help fill the prepared root canal. Zinc oxide, a powder, is mixed on a glass slab with liquid eugenol. The paste formed can be injected, placed with a spiral filler, applied with the file tip, or carried on the end of gutta-percha points into the canal (Fig. 4.91). When ZOE is used, a noneugenol base such as glass ionomer must be applied over the filling material before placement of the composite.

Noneugenol apical sealers include AH26 (Caulk, Milford, Delaware) and Diaket (Premier Dental, Norristown, Pennsylvania).

Calcium hydroxide is a temporary canal dressing supplied as a paste or powder. It is commonly used un-

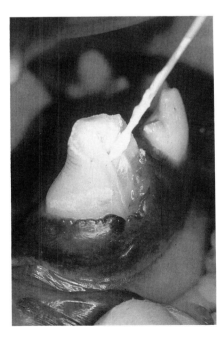

Fig. 4.91. Zinc oxide–eugenol sealing cement on gutta-percha.

der a restoration between the bonding material and gutta-percha. Calcium hydroxide also is used in the apexification process to stimulate hard tissue closure and in apexogenesis to help create a dentinal bridge.

In addition, calcium hydroxide is used to cover viable pulp in the vital pulpotomy procedure or dentin in indirect pulp capping. Calcium hydroxide protects the pulp by inducing formation of tertiary dentin. Calcium hydroxide has a limited shelf life because it reacts with carbon dioxide in the air. It must be kept in an airtight bottle. The surface layer of powder must be discarded before each use.

Sodium hypochlorite, or common household bleach, is the solution most frequently used to clean the root canal in conjunction with instrumentation in root canal therapy. It may be used as it comes from the bottle or diluted with one to two parts distilled water. This solution dissolves organic debris in the root canal.

SPECIAL CARE OF ENDODONTIC INSTRUMENTS
The endodontic file is flexible and extremely delicate. Should the instrument break within the root canal, apical surgery or extraction of the tooth may be necessary.

As instruments are prepared for sterilization, they must be individually checked for signs of wear, weakness, or fracture. If weakened or fractured, they must be discarded.

Restoratives

Restorations return teeth to as normal an appearance and function as possible. Amalgam, plastics, glass ionomer cements, semiprecious metals, and porcelain are commonly used restoratives.

Often, appearance and function conflict—restoring a tooth to normal size and color may not make it functional due to the inability of some restorations to hold up to repeated occlusal wear. In cases of conflict, function must prevail.

Amalgam is used to fill defects. Amalgam is inexpensive, strong, and resists wear. The mercury in amalgam is mixed with tin, copper, and zinc to create alloys. High copper amalgam alloys have increased strength and corrosion resistance. Unfortunately, commonly used amalgam does not bind to dentin or enamel, and it requires mechanical retention (undercuts). New amalgam bonding agents (Amalgabond by Parkell) preclude the need for undercutting and delineate marginal leakage.

Amalgam must be handled carefully to avoid operator contact with mercury. To keep mercury contamination at a minimum, purchase amalgam preencapsulated.

Disadvantages of using amalgam in veterinary dentistry include

- The need for additional equipment (an amalgamator) to mix encapsulated dental materials
- Marginal leakage
- Operator health precautions

  — Amalgam should never be touched with bare hands.
  — Masks must be worn and the work area well ventilated.

For reasons of safety, added working time, and the need for additional equipment, amalgam is not used as commonly as composite resins in the restoration process.

Glass ionomer cements are used as restoratives in the treatment of class two feline odontoclastic resorptive lesions, as an intermediate layer before acrylic restoration, for filling root canal access points in nonocclusal areas, and as a cement (Fig. 4.92).

Glass ionomer cements are classified as

- Type I (for cementing crowns, posts, orthodontic devices, and bridges)
- Type II (for restorations)
- Type III (for lining cements)
- Type IV (for fissure sealant)
- Type V (for orthodontic cements)
- Type VI (for core build-up cement)

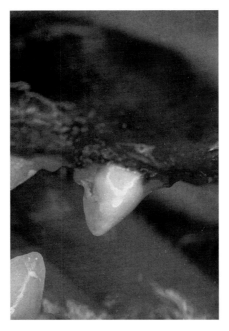

Fig. 4.92. Glass ionomer restoration of feline odontoclastic resorptive lesion.

Glass ionomer cements have many advantages:

- They slowly release fluoride, which decreases sensitivity, and have an antibacterial effect.
- They chemically bind with dentin and enamel.
- They mechanically bind with dentin.
- They can be applied in areas of slight moisture.

The main disadvantage of using glass ionomer cements for restorations is that they are less durable than other restoratives. Glass ionomer cements should not be placed on occlusal surfaces.

Glass ionomer cements come in various forms:

- **The nonencapsulated form**—Liquid and powder are mixed to a honeylike consistency with a spatula on a pad.

- **The encapsulated form**—This contains both powder and liquid. The capsules require an amalgamator and a special instrument to place the mixture.

- **The light-cured and self-cured forms**—The light-cured form requires a special light to induce polymerization. The self-cured form hardens in minutes.

The application of glass ionomer cements is different than that of composites and is technique sensitive.

- Prior to application of glass ionomer cement, the surface should not be bone dry.

- After the glass ionomer cement is applied, varnish, cocoa butter, or liquid light-cured resin is spread over the restoration surface to prevent moisture contamination. Once hardened, the restoration can be finished. Varnish is reapplied before the animal recovers from anesthesia.

DENTAL PLASTICS
Acrylics are powder and liquid combinations that form a hard plastic. Acrylics are used to make inclined planes for the movement of base narrow mandibular canine teeth (Fig. 4.93), as splints for fractured jaws, as temporary crowns, and as restoratives to fill access holes in endodontically treated teeth.

Dental plastics harden through polymerization. Once applied, the hardening process is initiated by mixing *A* material with *B* material (self-cured) or by applying an intense ultraviolet or visible light to the material (light-cured).

Self-cured composites will harden within minutes of mixture and must be applied to the restoration immediately (Fig. 4.94).

Light-cured composites allow the veterinarian an increased amount of time to place and shape the restoration before applying ultraviolet light for hardening. Curing time varies between 20 and 60 seconds depending on material used. When using a curing light, care should be taken by the operator not to look directly into the light source. Protective eyewear should be used.

> ⧠ **ADVANTAGES OF USING DENTAL PLASTICS**
> • Self-cured resins require no additional equipment.
> • They match the tooth color.
> • They can be polished.
> • Hybrid resins resist fracture and leakage.
>
> ⧠ **DISADVANTAGES OF USING DENTAL PLASTICS**
> • They are technique sensitive (and require multiple steps).
> • Light-cured resins require additional equipment.
> • Eugenol-containing materials (ZOE, gutta-percha) cannot be used in direct contact with composite resins.
> • They require mechanical retention (undercuts).
> • In time they will marginally leak.

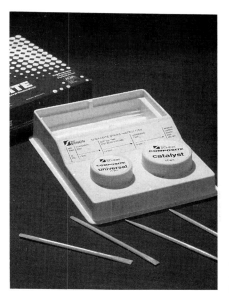

Fig. 4.94. Henry Schein self-cured composite kit.

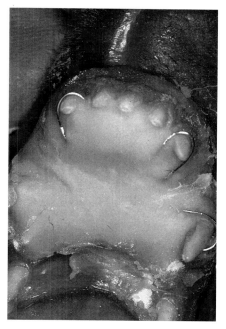

Fig. 4.93. Acrylic inclined bite plane used to correct base narrow canines.

Acrylic (composite) resins are used to restore teeth to normal appearance and function. Composites come in kits of liquids and semisolid materials that are mixed before application. They are classified according to the size of the filler and the type of curing employed (self or light).

• Type I resins are the pure, unfilled resins. They can be used as a cavity liner and are commonly employed with a filled resin (type II). Type I resins attach (bond) to clean, etched surfaces when applied in a thin film.

• Type II resins are filled to produce hardness and resistance to wear.

Proper type II composites must be chosen for a proposed application. Three types available include microfill, macrofill, and hybrid.

• **Microfilled** resins contain small particles that are easily polished. Microfilled resins fracture easily and must not be used on occlusal surfaces.

• **Macrofilled** composites wear well and can be used in stress-bearing areas. Their disadvantage is they are less polishable, which is of minimal concern when used on occlusal surfaces.

• **Hybrid** composites combine the polishability of the microfill resins and the fracture resistance of the macrofilled.

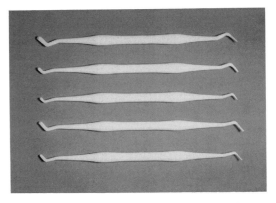

Fig. 4.95. Teflon instruments used to handle acrylic restoratives.

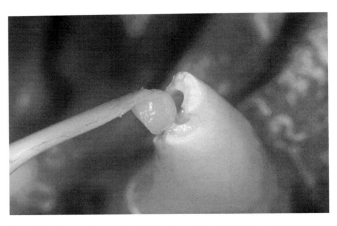

Fig. 4.96. Restorative applied to fracture site with Teflon instrument.

Bonding, also known as acid etch technique, is the physical adherence (sticking together) of one substance to another. This technique makes it possible to bond composite restorative materials directly to enamel and/or dentin (Figs. 4.95 and 4.96).

- **Enamel bonding** is accomplished by etching enamel to create a surface of microscopic undercuts. The restorative material penetrates into etched enamel and forms resin tags that mechanically interlock with the enamel surface. Only the enamel surface to be bonded to a restorative material is etched.

Etching solution (phosphoric acid) may be a liquid or gel. Etchant is applied to the enamel, allowed to sit for 30 seconds to one minute, then thoroughly rinsed and dried. Successful etching will produce a frosty white area.

- **Dentin bonding** differs from enamel bonding in that mechanical undercuts are not made. Dentin bonding employs chemical attachment. A liquid primer is brushed on the dentin surface and is not rinsed off.

- To bond with an **adhesive application**, the enamel is etched and the dentin primed, and then an adhesive is place before application of the composite.

Finishing and polishing the restoration are essential steps for creating a successful restoration. Fine finishing burs are used to contour and refine the restoration. Polishing stones and discs are used to complete the restoration.

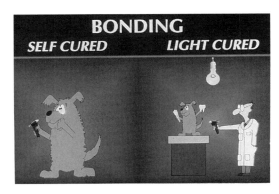

Fig. 4.97.

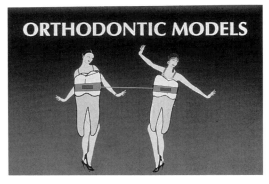

Fig. 4.98.

Orthodontic Materials

Alginate is impression material for orthodontic models (Fig. 4.98). A pastelike mixture of water and powder is prepared in a special green rubber bowl. The paste is poured onto a tray and compressed around the teeth for molding. The material hardens and may be removed after three minutes. Dental plaster and/or stone is poured into the impression to create a permanent model.

Dental plaster is a white powder that when mixed with water turns to paste that can be poured into an alginate impression. **Die stone**, also mixed with water, is harder than plaster and takes longer to harden. Die stone is poured first into the mold, followed by plaster. The alginate/plaster/stone combination is left undisturbed for a few hours, and then the alginate is removed, leaving a model of the teeth (Figs. 4.100 and 4.101).

Rubber-based impression material is used to make an accurate model of one or more teeth needed for crown or orthodontic fabrication. The material is either mixed by hand or loaded into a mixing syringe. Five minutes after injecting the mixed material around the tooth, the hardened impression can be removed and sent to the lab.

Brackets and **elastics** are used for tooth movement (Figs. 4.102–4.104). Frequently, dog and cat teeth are positioned in abnormal locations, causing trauma to other teeth and/or soft tissues. The placement of brackets, elastics, and arch wires often results in movement of the teeth into normal occlusion. Edgewise fixed or-

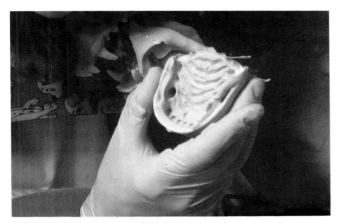

Fig. 4.99. Alginate impression of dog's maxilla.

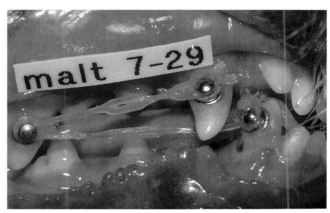

Fig. 4.102. Orthodontic brackets and elastics.

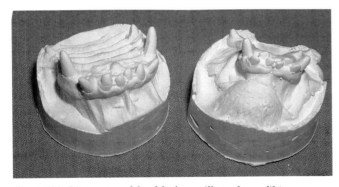

Fig. 4.100. Die stone models of dog's maxilla and mandible.

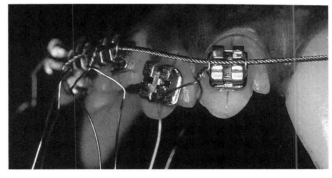

Fig. 4.103. Edgewise fixed orthodontic appliance.

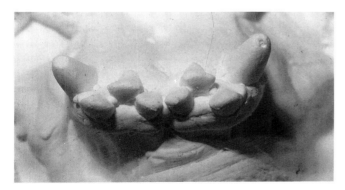

Fig. 4.101. Close-up detail of die stone model.

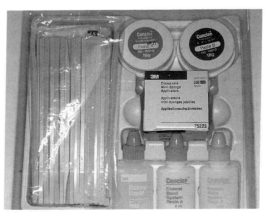

Fig. 4.104. Concise orthodontic bracket bonding kit.

thodontic appliances are brackets with rectangular slots attached to teeth and to a round or rectangular arch wire.

Dental Instruments and Materials by Procedure

Patient dental treatment cannot be interrupted for the lack of chairside instruments or materials. You must arm your technician with a list of instruments and materials needed for each procedure. Some examples:

- Prophy packet

  — Sickle scalers (H6/7, S6/7, N6/7, SH6/7)
  — Curettes (Gracey 12/13, Barnhart 5/6, Columbia 13/14)
  — Calculus-removing forceps. Its eccentric longer tip is placed over the crown and smaller tip under the ledge of calculus.
  — Periodontal probe/explorer
  — Polishing materials

- Tooth extraction

  — Number 15 blade
  — Blade handle
  — Suture material (2-0, 3-0, and 4-0 gut)
  — Forceps
  — Needle holders
  — Luxators
  — Root tip pick
  — Extraction forceps
  — Small scissors
  — Burs for high-speed drill (crosscut fissure and round)
  — Molt and Freer periosteal elevators

- Conventional endodontics

  — Round bur for access
  — K and H files
  — Barbed broaches
  — Gates Glidden drill (of appropriate size) loaded on slow speed handpiece with a 10:1 reduction gear
  — Sodium hypochlorite in 3-cc syringe
  — Gutta-percha points of appropriate lengths and widths
  — Zinc oxide-eugenol and glass slab spatula
  — College tipped applicator

  — Scissors
  — Plugger
  — Spreader
  — Touch 'n Heat
  — Inverted cone bur
  — Restoration packet
  — Glass ionomer cement

- Restoration packet

  — Z-100 kit
  — Light cure gun
  — Brushes
  — Acrylic tool
  — White stone bur on handpiece

- Vital pulpotomy packet

  — Retrograde amalgam carrier
  — Calcium hydroxide powder
  — Restoration packet
  — Round bur loaded on high-speed drill
  — Inverted cone bur

- Periodontal packet

  — Periodontal probe
  — Shepherd's hook explorer
  — Molt periosteal elevator (large and small)
  — Freer periosteal elevator
  — Ochsenbein chisel
  — Needle-holding forceps
  — Brown Adson forceps
  — Suture material (4-0 gut)
  — Curettes (Gracey 12/13, Barnhart 5/6, Columbia 13/14)
  — Number 3 pigtail explorer (for evaluating furcations)
  — Suture kit

- Orthodontic kit

  — Mouth trays (to pour alginate)
  — Alginate
  — Rubber mixing bowls
  — Wide spatula
  — Orthodontic cement (Concise)
  — Orthodontic buttons
  — Orthodontic brackets
  — Massel chain

5. THE WHY, WHEN, AND HOW OF SMALL ANIMAL DENTAL RADIOLOGY

Be not afraid of growing slowly; be afraid only of standing still.
—CHINESE PROVERB

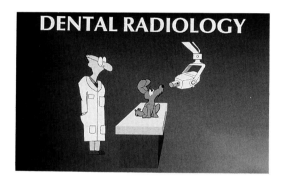

Fig. 5.1

After the physical exam, what is the first diagnostic tool you choose when presented an animal with a fractured limb? You take a radiograph. Why? To see what is hidden under the skin. The same premise must hold true for veterinary dentistry. In order to diagnose conditions and create a patient's dental treatment plan, the complete extent of existing pathology must be known. Radiology is essential in accessing this information.

Show your clients the films and, if the clients are at your clinic, their animals' pathology while the pets are anesthetized. If your clients cannot come to the clinic, consult with them by telephone and review the radiographs or Polaroid enlargements when the patients are released (Fig. 5.2). Inform your clients of proposed dental treatment and fees after radiographs are reviewed.

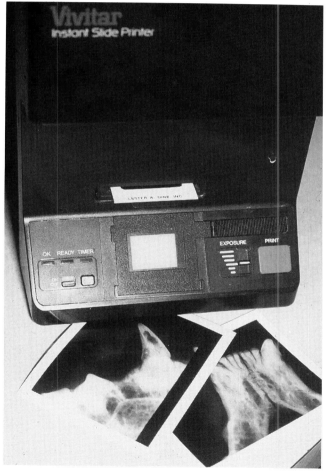

Fig. 5.2. Vivitar slide duplicator and Lester A. Dine film slide holder used to enlarge radiographs for client education.

WHY RADIOLOGY?

- To see pathology hiding below the gingiva or inside the teeth of cats and dogs (Figs. 5.3 and 5.4)
- To evaluate an area where the teeth are not apparent (Figs. 5.5 and 5.6)

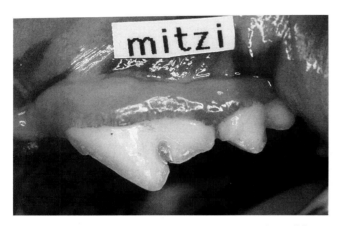

Fig. 5.3. Normal appearing left maxillary fourth premolar and first molar.

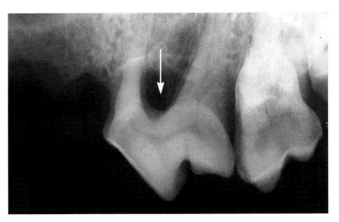

Fig. 5.4. Radiograph of teeth (Fig. 5.3), showing marked bone loss (arrow).

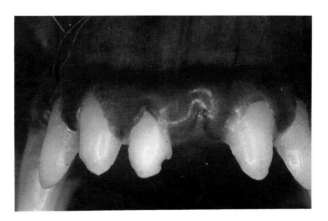

Fig. 5.5. Missing maxillary incisor.

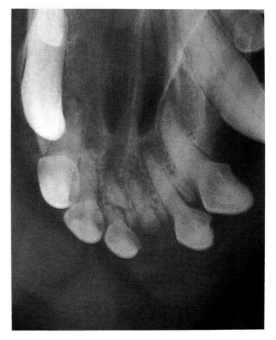

Fig. 5.6. Radiograph of maxillary incisors (Fig. 5.5), showing left central incisor retained root and fractured right central incisor.

- To document the obvious to support treatment decisions (Fig. 5.7)
- For client communication (Fig. 5.8)
- For medical/legal documentation
- For postoperative confirmation of proper extraction
- For preoperative, intraoperative, and postoperative endodontics (Figs. 5.9 and 5.10)
- To follow progression of pulpal pathology and/or periodontal disease
- For prepurchase exams on show dogs to see if the proper number of teeth exist

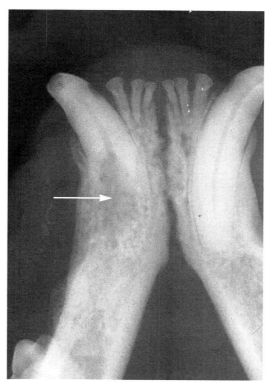

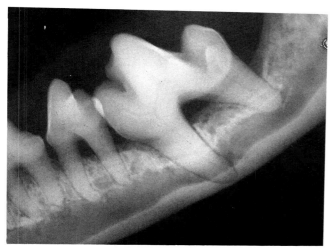

Fig. 5.7. Marked horizontal and vertical bone loss. Radiograph was taken prior to surgery to help in treatment planning.

Fig. 5.8. Radiograph of feline mandibular canine tooth fracture. The marked internal resorption of root apex (arrow) is used to explain to the client why the tooth cannot be saved endodontically.

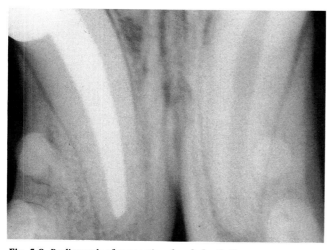

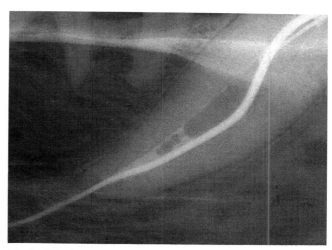

Fig. 5.9. Radiograph of conventional endodontic therapy.

Fig. 5.10. Radiograph of gutta-percha penetration through apex.

Periodontal disease is the most common ailment in small animals. Frequently, patients presented for "routine teeth cleaning and examination" have mobile teeth. The decision to extract, perform flap surgery, or provide only medical therapy is aided by radiographs, probe depths, and visual examination. The visual exam and probe depths are subjective tests, giving different results based on the examiner. Radiographs document the problem in black and white. The degree of bone loss can be measured, and radiographs provide permanent documentation of lesions.

The dental radiograph becomes part of your patient's permanent medical record. Examining serial radiographs of periodontal or endodontic cases radiographed at three- to six-month intervals provides invaluable information concerning progression or resolution of disease.

A radiograph also provides an opportunity to educate your pet owners about dental disease. A radiograph shows lesions above and below the gum line. It's one thing to tell a client that pathology exists, and a procedure should be performed, and quite another to show your client areas of bone loss around the tooth or a resorption that has "eaten away" the tooth's root. Seeing *is* believing.

Legal uses of radiographs to support treatment decisions prove invaluable. Without proof of endodontic disease or bone loss below the gingiva, a client may dispute dental therapy or the necessity of extractions.

WHEN TO TAKE A RADIOGRAPH

- When a tooth is mobile
- When gingiva bleeds with or without probing
- When a tooth is fractured
- When a tooth is discolored (pulpitis)
- When furcation exposure is present (periodontal disease)
- When teeth are missing without explanation
- When a feline odontoclastic resorptive lesion (FORL) is noted
- Prior to extraction for anatomical orientation and documentation

---

> **WHEN SHOULD FULL MOUTH (SIX VIEWS) RADIOGRAPHS BE TAKEN?**
> - When periodontal disease is present anywhere in the mouth
> - When feline odontoclastic resorptive lesions are diagnosed
> - If there are fractured teeth and the origin of the fracture is unknown
> - When evaluating the number of secondary teeth in a puppy or kitten as part of a soundness examination prior to purchase
> - To evaluate oral and facial swellings

HOW TO TAKE AN INTRAORAL RADIOGRAPH

The Radiograph Unit

Although the veterinarian has a choice to use his or her standard full body radiograph unit, delivery of *efficient* dental care necessitates the use of a dental radiograph unit. A dental radiology unit is a must in your dental operatory (Fig. 5.11).

From a dollars and cents standpoint, the dental radiograph unit is a profit center for the hospital. At least half of all teeth-cleaning patients need radiographic surveys. When radiographs are taken on all periodontal cases to evaluate degrees of bone loss, and when you respond by treating those cases with greater than 50

> **ADVANTAGES OF USING THE STANDARD WHOLE BODY VETERINARY RADIOLOGY UNIT**
> - No additional expense is necessary to purchase equipment.
> - Quality films can be exposed.
>
> **ADVANTAGES OF USING THE DENTAL RADIOGRAPH UNIT**
> - It is economical.
> - The extension arm varies in length, allowing vertical, horizontal, and rotational movement and necessitating less patient positioning.
> - The long arm can reach two closely located operatory areas.
> - Radiographs can be taken in the dental operatory rather than the patient having to be moved to the radiology area.
> - The shorter film focal length results in less scattered radiation.

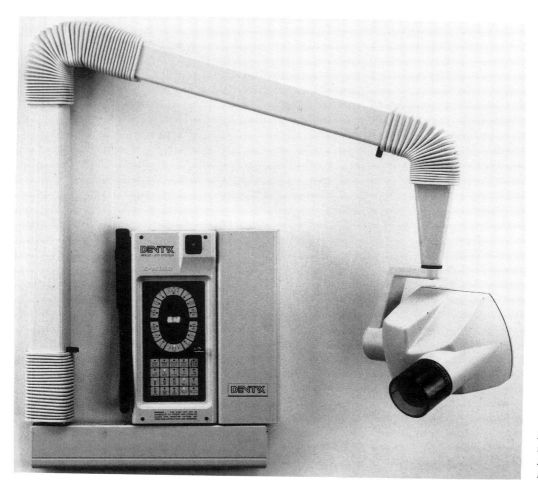

Fig. 5.11. Veterinary dental radiology unit (DentX Radiograph Unit, AFP Imaging Corporation).

percent bone loss, the dental radiograph unit will generate more additional practice income than any other piece of equipment. When the dental radiograph unit is used routinely, the $3000–$4000 invested in it will be paid back within three to six months of purchase.

ANATOMY OF A DENTAL RADIOGRAPH UNIT

The **position indicating device (PID)** is an extension cone placed on the tube head at the collimator attachment. To minimize the amount of radiation exposure, the PID is lead lined. The shape of the PID may be circular or rectangular. Rectangular-shaped PIDs limit the beam size to that of a number 2 periapical film.

The length of the PID provides an extension of 8, 12, or 16 in. from the radiograph tube to the animal's skin. The operator needs to decide which extension to use. Employing an 8-in. extension (using a 4-in. PID) is referred to as a **short cone technique** (Fig. 5.12), longer extensions result in a **long cone technique** (Fig. 5.13).

The short cone technique is preferable because it uses one-quarter the exposure, compared with the long cone technique, and is easier to position. The long cone technique produces films with increased detail.

The **arm** is the connection between the radiograph tube and control panel.

The **control panel** contains the timer and kilovoltage and/or milliamperage regulators (Fig. 5.14).

The **electric timer**, as a safety device, operates only while the switch is depressed and automatically cuts off the electric current at the end of the exposure. The timer resets itself after each exposure.

Most dental units use 110-v, 60-Hz AC electricity. A separate dedicated electrical circuit is recommended.

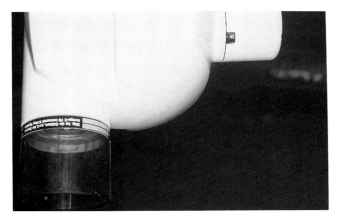

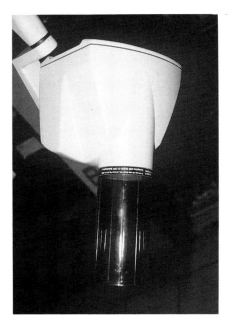

Fig. 5.12. *Short cone technique.*

Fig. 5.13. *Long cone technique.*

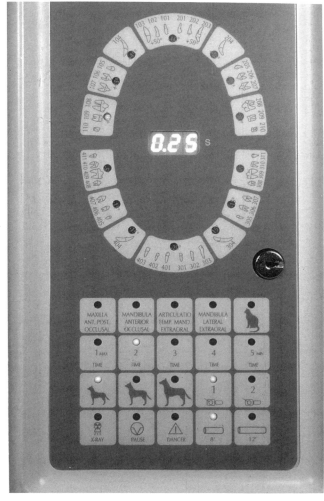

Fig. 5.14. *Control panel (DentX Radiograph Unit, AFP Imaging Corporation).*

RADIOGRAPH UNIT SETTINGS

Exposure variables considered in radiology include exposure time, kilovoltage peak, and milliamperes. Some units allow the operator to modify each variable based on the size of the patient and tooth type. Most units have one or two variables preset, allowing an operator to change exposure time.

> ❧ **EXPOSURE FACTORS AFFECTING FILM QUALITY**
> • kVp setting
> • mA setting
> • Exposure time setting
> • Film focal distance
> • Long or short cone

Kilovoltage peak (kVp) determines the quality of radiation produced. The higher the kVp setting, the higher the photon energy that strikes the tooth. Penetrating larger teeth requires a higher kilovoltage in order to get a diagnostic film. Most common kilovolt settings are from 50 to 100 kVp.

Speed (exposure time) is either measured in fractions of a second or pulses. A pulse is 1/60, or 0.016, of a second.

Milliamperes (mA) measure current and directly affect the number (quantity) of electrons. The milliampere number is set in most dental units between 7 and 15 mA. For standard veterinary radiograph units, 50 or 100 mA is commonly used. Changing the mA setting increases or decreases the intensity of the X-ray beam. *Increasing the mA increases the density of the radiograph.*

Film focal distance (FFD) is another important variable. Moving the tube closer or farther away from the patient can affect the intensity of the X-ray beam. As the distance from the patient is decreased (short cone technique), intensity of the radiation reaching the patient increases. As the distance is increased, intensity of the radiation reaching the patient is decreased (long cone technique).

CONE LENGTH
Dental radiograph unit cones come in a variety of sizes, from 4 to 16 in. Exposure adjustments must be made depending on the size used. For example, a 4-in. cone would require one-quarter of the exposure needed by an 8-in. cone.

The PID is placed against the patient's maxilla or mandible. This results in an FFD of 8, 12, or 16 in., depending on the cone length. For a standard veterinary radiograph unit, the tube head (without a cone) is placed 12–16 in. away from the tooth.

TOOTH FILM DISTANCE
In the intraoral technique, film is placed parallel to the palatal or lingual tooth surface. Due to the size of small animal oral anatomy, this is not always possible. Instead, a **bisecting angle technique** is used, resulting in a 20- to 50-degree angulation of the X-ray beam to the film plane, depending on which tooth is radiographed.

> ⊙ **RULES FOR SUCCESSFUL POSITIONING FOR DENTAL RADIOGRAPHS**
> • The closer the object being radiographed is to the film, the sharper and more accurate the image.
> • Use the longest film focal distance practical.
> • Direct the central beam as close to a right angle (or bisecting angle) to the film as possible.
> • Maintain as parallel an interface between the film and object as possible.

DIGITAL IMAGING DENTAL RADIOLOGY
Digital imaging is a recent technical advancement in dental radiology (Fig. 5.15). It will be as popular as, or even replace, film-based imaging in the future.

Computer image capturing and image enhancement has many advantages compared with the traditional film systems. With digital imaging, the dental radiograph unit is still used to expose the lesion, but instead of film, a sensor pad is placed inside the mouth and accepts the image and transfers it to the computer screen (Fig. 5.16). Advantages over the traditional film-based systems include

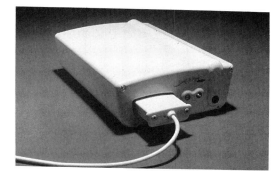

Fig. 5.15. Dental digital imaging unit (Sens-a-Ray, AFP Imaging Corporation).

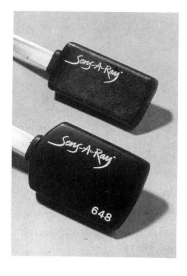

Fig. 5.16. Digital imaging sensors (Sens-a-Ray, AFP Imaging Corporation).

• A 75–90 percent reduction in radiation is needed to produce an image.

• There is instant image production—no processing with chemicals.

• You can retake film immediately if you are not pleased with the image.

• You are able to enlarge the entire image or a certain section, to adjust contrast and brightness, to enhance the margins, and to rotate images (Fig. 5.17).

• You can measure distances between two points, which helps in estimating endodontic working file lengths (Fig. 5.18).

• You can measure tooth densities for evaluation of areas of decreased density (class one or two feline odontoclastic resorptive lesions).

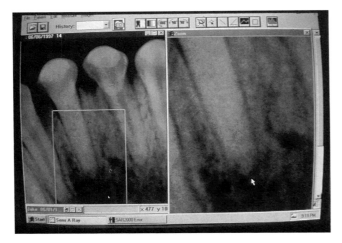

Fig. 5.17. Digital imaging picture and enlargement.

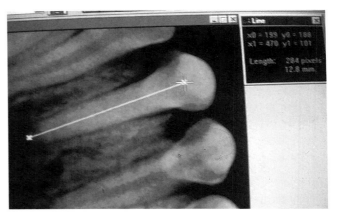

Fig. 5.18. Digital length measurement of root canal for endodontic therapy.

Radiation Safety

THE ALARA PRINCIPLE

ALARA stands for as low as reasonably achievable. This concept endorses the use of the lowest-possible exposure of the patient (and operator) to radiation to produce a diagnostically acceptable radiograph.

Staff of the veterinary facility must be protected against radiation exposure.

Shielding of the X-ray beam in the unit greatly reduces occupational exposure. Lead aprons must be worn at all times when taking films.

VETERINARIAN RESPONSIBILITIES

- Prescribe only those radiographs that are diagnostically necessary.

- Install and maintain radiographic equipment in safe working condition.

- Use minimum exposure E speed film if possible; however, the D ultraspeed is most commonly used in veterinary medicine.

- All personnel who expose radiographs must be adequately trained, supervised, and monitored.

- General anesthesia is mandatory for any radiographed animal. Total immobilization allows the technician to position radiograph film in the patient's mouth without exposing his or her hands to radiation.

There are three types of radiation—primary, secondary, and leakage.

- **Primary radiation** comes from direct exposure to the X-ray beam. The operator must always keep away from the primary beam of the radiograph unit. The veterinarian or staff should never hold films in the patient's mouth with bare or gloved fingers. Devices must be used to position the film in the mouth without operator exposure.

- **Secondary (scatter) radiation** comes from areas that have been irradiated by the primary beam. Protective aprons must be worn to help shield the body from this type of radiation.

- **Leakage radiation** comes from the tube housing and not the primary beam. Neither the tube housing nor the cone should be held during exposure.

PERSONNEL MONITORING

A film badge monitoring service is used to provide radiation monitoring for all members of the office staff functioning near the film exposure. The **dosimeter badge** is worn at all times in the veterinary office. It measures the amount and type of radiation an individual is exposed to in the working environment. The badge should not be worn outside of the office.

For the office staff a monthly report on radiation monitoring should be a permanent record and should be saved indefinitely.

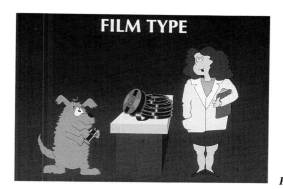

Fig. 5.19.

Film

Small intraoral film is used in dental radiography. It is inexpensive, flexible, and provides great detail. Nonscreen film is preferable due to the high definition necessary to interpret dental lesions. Dental film is conveniently used for intra- or extraoral placement.

Individual dental film is packaged in a light-tight packet that is made of either plastic or paper (Fig. 5.20). Inside the packet, film is positioned between an inner lining of two sheets of black paper. A sheet of lead foil is located at the "back" of the packet, next to the tab opening. Lead foil protects the film from secondary radiation, which may cause the film to fog.

The back of the packet has a tab opening used to remove film for processing. This side is placed next to the tongue or palate.

Intraoral dental film is packaged with one or two films per packet. When two films are exposed, the practitioner may give the second film to the client or referring veterinarian. Film packets are color coded—green indicates a single-film packet, and gray a two-film packet.

FILM SPEED
Commonly used dental film is available as **speed D** (ultraspeed) and **speed E** (ekta speed). Speed E film is rated at twice the speed of D film and requires half the exposure time, with a moderate loss of quality. In veterinary dentistry, speed D is predominantly used due to its better quality.

FILM SIZES
Three sizes of dental film are frequently used in veterinary dentistry (Fig. 5.21):

• Child periapical size 0 measures $7/8 \times 1^5/8$ in. It's used mostly in cats, exotics, and small dogs.

• Adult periapical size 2, also called standard size, measures $1^1/4 \times 1^9/16$ in. Size 2 is the most popular size used.

• Occlusal size 4 measures $2^1/4 \times 3$ in. Occlusal film is used to radiograph larger teeth and for survey studies.

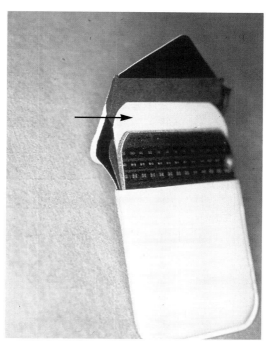

Fig. 5.20. Film packet contents (arrow points to the film).

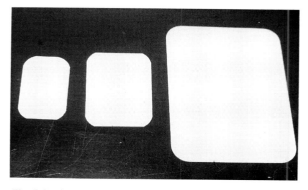

Fig. 5.21. (From left to right) *Sizes 0, 2, and 4 film.*

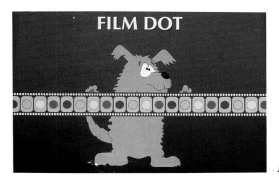

Fig. 5.22.

FILM DOT

Dental film is embossed with a raised dot in one of the corners. The convex side of the dot indicates the front side of the film. The dot is used to identify the right side of the mouth from the left (Figs. 5.23 and 5.24). *The convex (raised) dot is placed at the occlusal edge and toward the radiograph tube.*

To determine whether a film is on the right or left side, observe where the convex dot is located and identify the progression of teeth from incisors to molars. *Hint:* mentally place the film in your mouth and imagine the dot orientation and progression of premolars to molars to help determine if the film is on the right or left side of the mouth.

FILM MOUNTING

After films are processed and dried, they are mounted in cardboard or plastic holders (Fig. 5.25). Mounting makes films easy to view, allows patient identification, and protects film from damage.

Mounts are labeled with the patient's name and the date of the study. The films are laid out so the embossed dots are located in the upper left corner. Maxillary films are positioned above the mandibular films. Mount the films with the raised portion of the dot toward you. Read films as if you were facing your patient.

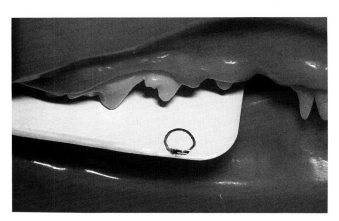

Fig. 5.23. Film dot next to right maxillary premolars.

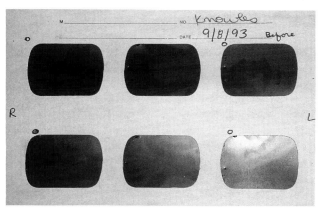

Fig. 5.25. Film mounts.

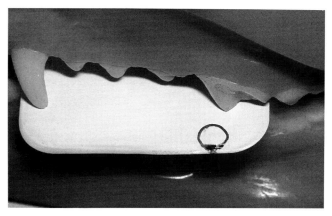

Fig. 5.24. Film dot next to left maxillary premolars.

RADIOGRAPHIC LANDMARKS

It is important to be able to look at a film and identify the area exposed.

- **Maxillary incisors**—Look for a large radiodense (white area) distal to the teeth, with two ovals representing the palative fissures (Fig. 5.26). All incisor teeth have one root.

- **Mandibular incisors**—Look for a radiolucent black space separating the mandibular rami (Fig. 5.27).

- **Maxillary premolars and molars**—Look for a fine white line representing the maxillary recess apical to the roots (Fig. 5.28).

- **Mandibular premolars and molars**—Look for radiolucent (black areas) above and below the jaw (Fig. 5.29). Other than the first premolar (in the dog), all mandibular premolars and molars have two roots.

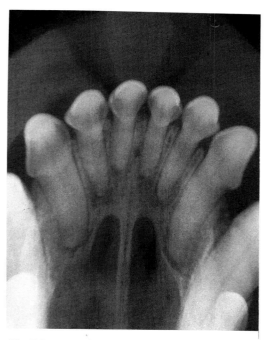

Fig. 5.26. Maxillary incisors.

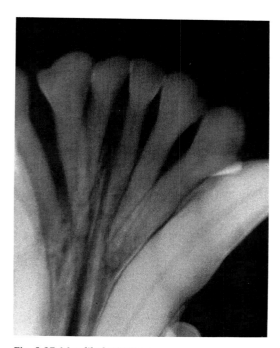

Fig. 5.27. Mandibular incisors.

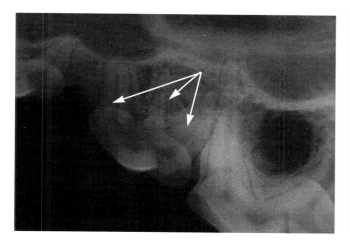

Fig. 5.28. Maxillary premolars and molars. Note abnormal, triple-rooted third premolar (arrows).

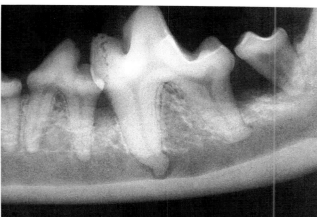

Fig. 5.29. Mandibular premolars and molars.

POSITIONING THE FILM AND PATIENT

Place film inside the mouth, parallel to the teeth to be examined. Film is held in position by the endotracheal tube, wadded up newspaper, lead radiograph gloves (without fingers inside), sponges, clay encased in a plastic bag, or commercial holding devices (Fig. 5.30). The operator must not use his or her fingers to hold film to be exposed.

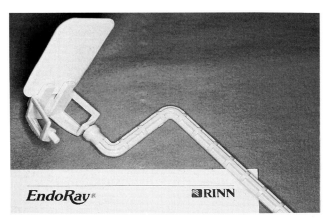

Fig. 5.30. Rinn film-holding device.

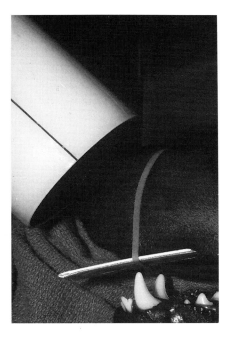

Fig. 5.31. Anterior maxillary film and PID position.

Immobilization of the patient is essential to image sharpness. Movement of the film packet or the patient's head must be avoided during exposure. Vibration and other movement of the radiograph tube will cause a blurred image.

Due to the size of small animal oral anatomy, the **bisecting angle technique** is used in most exposures. Lay film far enough inside the animal's mouth so that the tooth's root structure will be projected onto the film. Imaginary lines are drawn along the long axis of the tooth and the plane of the film. The point where these two lines meet will create an angle. Instead of the central beam being aimed perpendicular to the film as in the parallel technique, the central beam is aimed perpendicular to the line bisecting the angle created between the line of the tooth and the line of the film.

Angulation of the primary beam is dependent on which area is being radiographed.

Anterior maxilla: The patient indicator device (PID) is aimed at the root apex of the first premolar at a 45-degree angle rostral to the hard palate (Fig. 5.31).

Maxillary cheek teeth: The PID is aimed at the root apex of the fourth premolar at 45 degrees and is pointed toward the palate (Figs. 5.32 and 5.33).

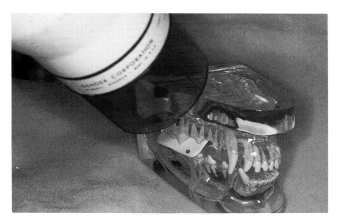

Fig. 5.32. Maxillary premolar film and PID position. Note location of film dot.

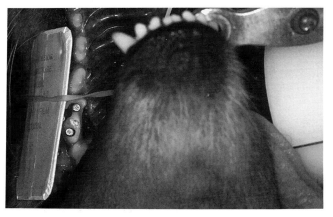

Fig. 5.33. Extraoral film and PID position of maxillary cheek teeth.

Anterior mandible: The PID is aimed at the root apex of the first premolar at –20 degrees to the ventral border of the mandible (Fig. 5.34).

Mandibular cheek teeth: Anterior—PID is aimed at the root apex of the first premolar at 45 degrees (Fig. 5.35). Posterior—PID is aimed at 90 degrees to the tooth.

Vertical angulation refers to the up and down movement of the PID. Vertical angulation will determine how accurately the length of the object being radiographed is reproduced.

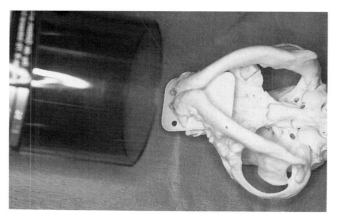

Fig. 5.34. Anterior mandibular incisors film and PID position.

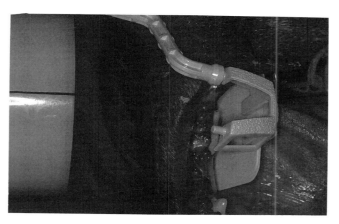

Fig. 5.35. Mandibular premolar and molar film and PID position.

FORESHORTENED IMAGE

Changes in vertical angulation are similar to those changes in shadows caused by the earth rotating around the sun. At noon, when the sun is directly overhead, a shadow is **foreshortened** (shorter). Foreshortened images appear shorter than the subjects really are, the result of too much vertical angulation. To normalize a foreshortened image, the vertical angulation is reduced (Figs. 5.36–5.39).

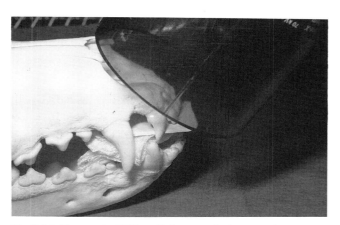

Fig. 5.36. Placement of PID at 45 degrees to incisors, resulting in bisected angle image.

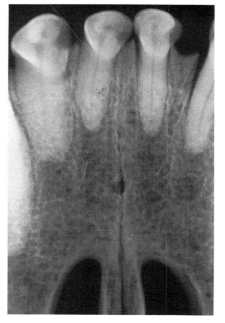

Fig. 5.37. Normal image of maxillary incisors.

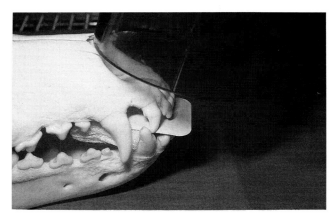

Fig. 5.38. Placement of PID at 80 degrees to incisors, resulting in foreshortened image.

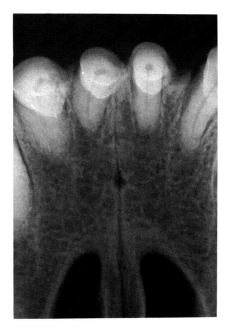

Fig. 5.39. Foreshortened image.

ELONGATED IMAGE

In late afternoon, as the sun nears the horizon, shadows are **elongated** (lengthened). Elongated images appear longer than the subjects really are, the result of too little vertical angulation. An elongated image of a tooth will make it appear longer than the anatomical length (Figs. 5.40 and 5.41). To correct an elongated image, vertical angulation is increased.

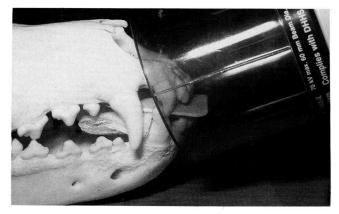

Fig. 5.40. Placement of PID at 20 degrees, resulting in elongated image.

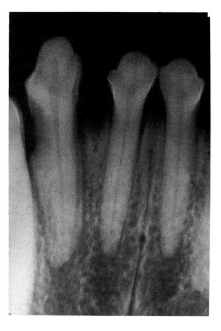

Fig. 5.41. Elongated image.

Horizontal angulation refers to back and forth movements on a plane that is parallel with the floor. Proper horizontal angulation produces normal interproximal anatomic representation of the teeth without teeth overlapping.

Horizontal (paralleling) technique directs the central beam at right angles to the tooth and film. When a single tooth is radiographed, the film packet is placed parallel to the long axis of the tooth. With the horizontal technique, the central beam is projected at a right angle to the film packet. In the dog and cat, this is accomplished best when radiographing mandibular cheek teeth.

"SLOB" RULE

When two roots of a triple-rooted tooth are superimposed on the radiograph, it is difficult to evaluate both roots. In order to visualize the roots, two radiographs are taken at oblique angles. Vertical position is fixed, and the tube is moved horizontally. Horizontal tube shift will result in a film with the overlapped roots moved apart. When the root "moves" in an opposite direction to the horizontal shift of the tube, then the root is labial or buccal. If the root "moves" in the same direction as the tube, it is lingual or palatal. SLOB stands for "same lingual, opposite buccal."

Film Processing

Proper exposure of film is only one of the steps in producing quality dental radiographs. Processing the film completes the procedure.

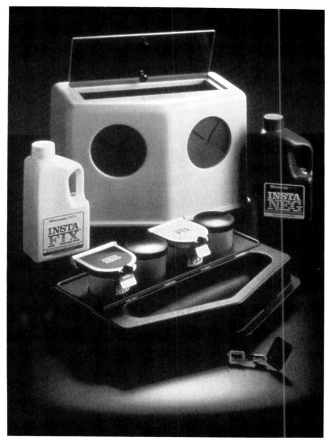

Fig. 5.42. Insta-veloper Portable Darkroom: chairside developer with developer, water, and fixer in separate containers. Courtesy of Microcopy.

> ☞ PROCESSING FUNDAMENTALS
> • Active, fresh processing solutions
> • A standardized method of processing
> • A light-secured area

Film may be developed

• By hand with regular or rapid dental-processing solutions in the darkroom

• With the chairside developer, a portable, light-safe box with developer, fixer, and water in small containers (Figs. 5.42 and 5.43). The operator places his or her hands through two diaphragms in a lighted room to access the solutions. The box's top, an orange or red Plexiglas safety filter, enables the operator to see inside. The whole process, from opening the film packet to examination of a rinsed film, takes approximately one minute.

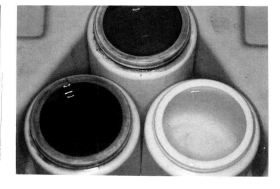

Fig. 5.43. Close-up of developing solutions.

• Automatically. Film is placed into one end of the automatic dental processor and comes out fully developed, fixed, and dried in two to seven minutes. Using a standard veterinary automatic processor is discouraged because small dental films may become lost in the processor, and tape used to attach the dental films to larger films may harm the processor's rollers.

• Quickly in the film packet (Veterinary Dental Film System [VDFS], Hawaii Mega-cor, Inc., Aiea, Hawaii). Film is developed in 30 seconds within the film packet after infusion of developer and fixer solutions (Fig. 5.44).

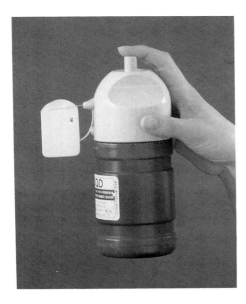

Fig. 5.44. Processing of instant dental radiograph.

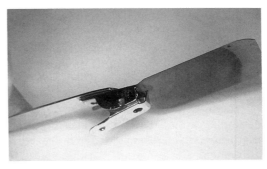

Fig. 5.45. Film clip with film attached.

To produce radiographs of good quality, processing solutions must be fresh. Solution containers are covered at all times to minimize evaporation. The maximum effective lifetime of the processing solutions varies with use. One rule is, with routine use, to change solutions every other week. If many films are processed, solutions become exhausted and need replacement more often.

Quality Control

A good radiograph is useless unless it is read accurately, and a poor radiograph cannot be read properly.

A quality assurance film should be exposed daily to verify that all parts of the dental radiography system are working properly. The use of a **step wedge** helps accomplish this goal (Fig. 5.46). The step wedge is an object composed of several graduated pieces of aluminum placed so that each successive piece is shorter, thus producing a step effect.

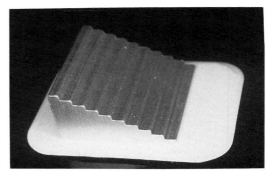

Fig. 5.46. Step wedge placed on top of number 2 film.

STEPS FOR MANUALLY PROCESSING DENTAL RADIOGRAPHS

• Once the film packet is in a light-secured area, open the packet tab and slide forward the paper liner and film. This will reveal the film to be processed. Only touch the sides of the film with your fingers.
• Attach a film hanger to the film (Fig. 5.45). The film should extend horizontally from the clip. Give the film a gentle tug to make certain it is firmly attached to the clip.
• Place the film into the developing solution for 10–30 seconds. (Leave film in solution longer if the room temperature is less than 68°F.)
• Rinse the film in distilled water for 10 seconds.
• Place the film in the fixing solution for 30 seconds.
• Rinse for 30 seconds in distilled water.
• After viewing, place the film in the fixer for 5 minutes and rinse in distilled water for 20 minutes.
• When rinsing is complete, hang radiograph on a rack to dry or use a hair drier for rapid drying.

USE OF THE STEP WEDGE TO ESTABLISH A CONTROL RADIOGRAPH

• Dental film is laid tab side down on a flat surface.
• A step wedge is placed over the film.
• Expose as if you were taking a radiograph of a 25-lb dog's canines.
• Process using new chemicals.

The processed image ideally shows 10 shades of varying densities from light gray to black (Fig. 5.47). If all 10 steps are not apparent, adjust exposure up or down until all can be distinctly seen. If the lightest steps (from the thickest part of the wedge) are indistinct, increase the exposure. If the darkest steps (from the thinnest part of the wedge) are indistinct, decrease the exposure. Once the correct exposure is determined, this becomes the **control film**. Expose, but do not develop, 20–30 films.

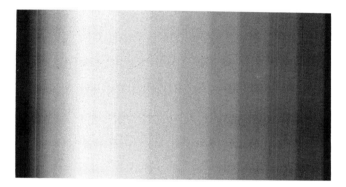

Fig. 5.47. Step wedge radiograph processed in fresh developing solutions.

DAILY QUALITY CONTROL USING STEP WEDGE RADIOGRAPHS

Mount the control film processed with new solutions next to the view box. Every two or three days, process a test film and compare it with the control film. If they are not identical, verify that the processing time and temperature were correct. If more than two steps are lighter than those in the control film, the processing solutions are exhausted and need changing (Fig. 5.48).

Fig. 5.48. Step wedge radiograph processed in exhausted developing solutions.

Film quality encompasses many variables:

- **Density** is the degree of blackness created on the radiograph film. Density is controlled by milliampere-seconds (mAs). Ten to 12.5 mAs will provide good detail.

- **Contrast** is the relative difference between densities. High-contrast film would include areas of white and black. Low-contrast films may appear gray. Contrast is controlled by kilovoltage peak (kVp), which is normally between 50 and 90, and processing variables (such as temperature, development time, and light leaks).

- The range of development times is related to the solution temperature recommended by the manufacturer. **Underdevelopment** (caused by weak, exhausted, cold solutions or by too short a development time) results in poor contrast. **Overdevelopment** causes fog and overall darkening of the image.

TROUBLESHOOTING REASONS FOR POOR FILM QUALITY

Faulty radiographs are commonly caused by

- Incorrect positioning of the film packet or tube head
- Incorrect processing procedures
- Incorrect kilovoltage
- Movement of the patient or tube head during the exposure

Film fogging appears as a gray or dark film (Fig. 5.49). Causes include

- Film not being placed in fixer long enough. This is the most common reason for film fogging and is easy to diagnose and repair: immerse the film into the fixer for another five minutes to see if the image improves.
- Exhausted processing chemicals
- Outdated film
- Light leaks in film packet
- Overprocessing (placing the film in the developer too long or in too hot a developing solution)
- Film processed in fixer-contaminated developer
- Film exposed to stray radiation, excessive heat, or light leaking into processing area

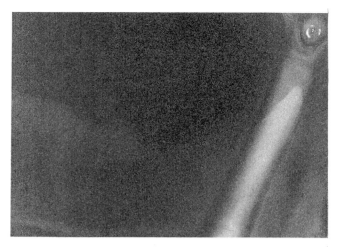

Fig. 5.49. Film fogging.

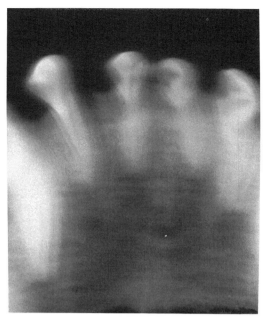

Fig. 5.50. Blurred image.

No image is the result of

- The film being immersed in the fixer before the developer
- The film not being exposed at all, if it is completely clear

Light film is the result of

- Not enough exposure time
- Not enough kilovoltage
- Weak developer
- Too short a time in developer solution

Causes of **dark film** include

- Too high a kilovoltage
- Too much exposure time
- Film processed too long in developing solution
- Developing solution being too warm (the ideal temperature is 68°F)

A **blurred image** results from motion during exposure (Fig. 5.50). The patient, film, or radiograph head moved.

A **partial image** (Fig. 5.51) is caused by

- Film being partially immersed in developer
- Film in the developer coming into contact with other films or the side of the tank
- The film or tube head being incorrectly positioned

Fingerprints come from poor handling (Fig. 5.52). Film must be touched only on the edges.

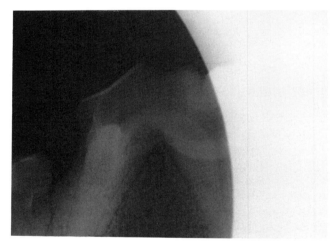

Fig. 5.51. Partial image.

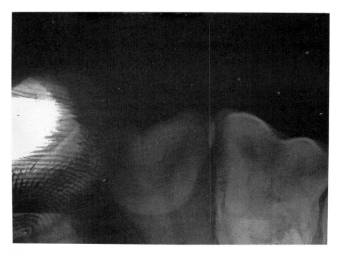

Fig. 5.52. Fingerprints on processed film.

Normally, a finished, dry film will be smooth and shiny. When film is not washed thoroughly, or rinsed in water mixed with fixer, the fixer will dry on the film, leaving a frosty finish. **Frosty-appearing film** is a common problem that is easily prevented by using fresh distilled water with each study.

Streaked film is film that was insufficiently developed, fixed, or rinsed or was processed in contaminated solutions.

Crescent-shaped lines result when the film packet is sharply bent, damaging the film (Fig. 5.53).

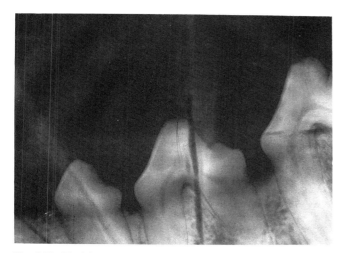

Fig. 5.53. Black line in center of film is due to bent film packet.

> ☙ **COMMON CAUSES FOR POOR QUALITY FILMS**
> • Incorrect film positioning
> • Movement of tube head or patient during exposure
> • Incorrect exposure setting
> • Placing film backwards in mouth
> • Exposing film twice
> • Poor processing

A WORTHY GOAL
The dental technician should be able to expose and process a full set of diagnostic intraoral films (six) within 20 minutes.

INTERPRETING DENTAL RADIOGRAPHS

The radiograph, when correlated with the pet's case history and a clinical examination, is one of the most important diagnostic aids available to the veterinarian. When examined under proper conditions, dental radi-ographs of diagnostic quality reveal evidence of disease that cannot be found in any other way.

Be careful, however, not to confuse some normal anatomical structures with pathology (Fig. 5.54).

- The middle mental foramen, the opening in the mandible through which the mental nerve passes, is located ventral to the mandibular first or second premolar near the root apex of the canine tooth.

- The posterior mental foramen is located ventral to the mandibular third premolar. At times, it can be confused with a periapical lesion. If in doubt, radiograph the tooth at an oblique angle, which will show the foramen not connected to the tooth's apex.

- The mandibular canal, located on the ventral border of the mandible, may be superimposed on apices of mandibular cheek teeth and appear to be periapical disease.

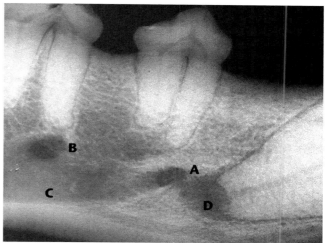

Fig. 5.54. Radiograph showing middle mental foramen (A), posterior mental foramina (B), mandibular canal (C), and periapical endodontic lesion (D).

Radiology of Periodontal Disease

The most common disease in small animals older than five years is periodontal disease. Treatment may include supragingival and subgingival scaling, periodontal surgery, tooth resection, or tooth extraction. Radiography plays an important role in determining the extent of periodontal disease and helps dictate therapy. When evaluating periodontal disease, the clinician uses radiographs to evaluate the following:

- Alveolar bone changes
- Interdental bone height
- Presence of the lamina dura, the bone lining the tooth socket
- Trabecular patterns
- Size of periodontal ligament space
- Degree of bone loss

A radiograph shows a two-dimensional representation of a three-dimensional structure and may not adequately represent the severity of disease. Early destructive bone lesions sometimes are not radiographically observable. Buccal and lingual alveolar bone are particularly difficult to evaluate because they are superimposed. In addition to radiographic findings, the clinician must rely on clinical examination of sulcular depths, tooth mobility, and appearance of attached gingiva in order to decide on the diagnosis and treatment plan.

Normal, healthy alveolar bone has a characteristic appearance on radiographs. The alveolar crest is situated approximately 1 to 2 mm apical to the cemento-enamel junction (CEJ) of the teeth of cats and dogs. The shape of the alveolar crest may vary from rounded to flat. Between incisor teeth, the alveolar crest will usually appear pointed. Between premolar and molar teeth, the crest will be parallel to a line between the adjacent CEJs where the enamel thins and disappears.

The alveolar crest is continuous with the lamina dura of adjacent teeth (Fig. 5.55). When lamina dura and periodontal ligaments are examined, only interproximal portions are visible. Buccal and lingual areas are not seen in the radiograph.

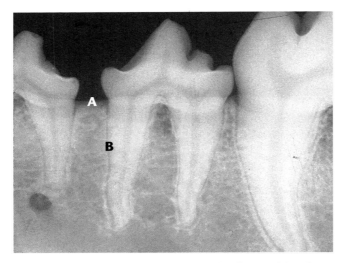

Fig. 5.55. Radiograph of normal appearing alveolar crest (A) *and lamina dura* (B).

BONE CHANGES DETECTED BY RADIOLOGY
Crestal Lamina Dura
Normally, a radiopaque line covers the alveolar socket and extends on top of interdental bone. Because the facial and lingual bony plates are obscured by dense root structure, radiographic evaluation of bone changes in periodontal disease is based mainly on the interdental septa.

With marked periodontal disease, crestal lamina dura is indistinct, irregular, fuzzy, and radiolucent. Widening of the periodontal ligament space and loss of lamina dura are due to resorption of the alveolar bone secondary to periodontal disease.

Bone Level
Normally, the crest of interdental bone appears 1–2 mm below the cemento-enamel junction in cats and dogs. Bone level in periodontal disease is lowered as inflammation extends and bone is resorbed.

The overall height of alveolar crestal bone in relationship to the cemento-enamel junction is used to evaluate bone loss. Distribution of bone loss is classified as either **localized** or **generalized** depending on the number of areas affected. Localized bone loss occurs in isolated areas; generalized bone loss involves the majority of the crestal bone.

Initially, periodontitis develops as a localized erosion of the alveolar crest. Bony changes cannot be radiographically detected until they are advanced. As the severity of periodontitis increases, more alveolar bone is destroyed, and the process becomes generalized.

Periodontal Ligament Space
The periodontal ligament is composed of connective tissue. It normally appears as a fine radiolucent line next to the root surface. On its outer side is lamina dura, bone lining the tooth socket, which appears radiopaque.

When examining a radiograph for periodontal disease, the lamina dura of each tooth is inspected to see if it is continuous or breached, indicating pathology. Absence of the lamina dura and lack of continuity are indicative of periodontal disease. With disease, the periodontal ligament space may appear of varying thickness, indicating disease involvement is not consistent around the entire root. Usually teeth with marked periodontal spaces are mobile.

Patterns of Bone Loss
The interdental septa may be reduced in height with the crest horizontal and perpendicular to the long axis of the adjacent teeth, or there may be vertical (angular) bone loss. A reduction of only 1 mm in the thickness of the cortical plate is sufficient to permit radiographic visualization.

Amount of Bone Loss

Radiography is an indirect method for determining the amount of bone loss in periodontal disease. It shows the amount of remaining bone rather than the amount lost.

STAGES OF PERIODONTAL DISEASE

Gingivitis

Periodontal disease is classified from stages one to four based on the severity of radiographic and clinical signs. Stage one is referred to as early gingivitis. Clinically, the gingiva appears inflamed. In stage one disease, there is no bone loss.

Stage two, or advanced gingivitis, is typified by inflammation and swelling. There are still no radiographic changes observable.

Early Periodontitis

The earliest radiographic sign of periodontitis is a loss of definition in the crestal bone (Fig. 5.56). The alveolar crest loses its distinct sharp appearance and becomes blunted. Bony margins become diffuse and irregular and may show areas of localized erosion. In the incisor regions, there is blunting of the alveolar crests. In the premolar and molar regions, there may also be loss of normally sharp angles between the lamina dura and the alveolar crests.

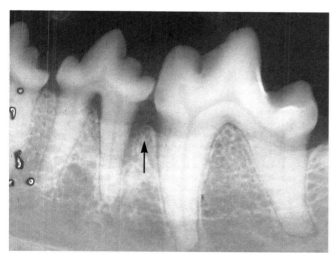

Fig. 5.56. Radiograph of early periodontitis. Note loss of alveolar crest (arrow).

Established Periodontitis

Stage three periodontal disease is typified by pocket formation. Radiographically, bony destruction extends to the buccal and/or lingual alveolar plates. There may also be horizontal or vertical defects.

Horizontal bone loss radiographically appears as decreased alveolar bone around several adjacent teeth (Figs. 5.58 and 5.59). Crestal bone is normally located

1 mm apical to the cemento-enamel junction in dogs and cats. With horizontal bone loss, both the buccal and lingual plates of bone as well as interdental bone have been resorbed. A **suprabony pocket** exists where the epithelial attachment is above the bony defect and is associated with horizontal bone loss.

Horizontal bone loss may be classified as localized or generalized, depending on the regions involved, and as mild (less than 10 percent bone loss), moderate (10–30 percent), or severe (greater than 30 percent), depending on the extent of bone loss.

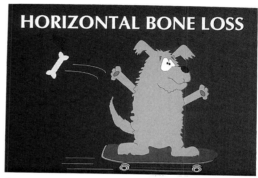

Fig. 5.57.

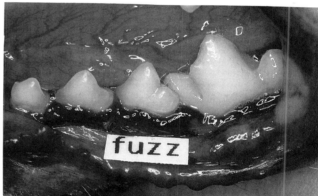

Fig. 5.58. Normal appearing gingiva.

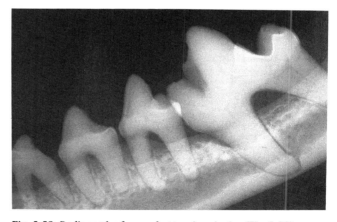

Fig. 5.59. Radiograph of normal appearing gingiva (Fig. 5.58) revealing marked horizontal bone loss in dog on long-term steroids for allergic dermatitis.

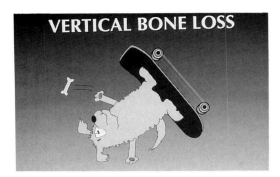

VERTICAL BONE LOSS

Fig. 5.60.

Vertical bone defects are also called **infrabony** (or **intrabony**) defects (Figs. 5.61 and 5.62). The epithelial attachment on the root surface is below the crest of bone. Infrabony lesions are classified by the number of walls remaining. The defect extends apically from the alveolar crest and is initially surrounded by three walls of bone: two marginal (lingual or palatal and facial) and a hemisepta (the bone of the interdental septum that remains on the root of the uninvolved adjacent tooth). As disease progresses, two, one, or no (cup) walled defects may occur.

Radiographically, a vertical bone defect is generally V shaped and sharply outlined. It is immediately adjacent to the root surface of the affected tooth, and the adjacent bone has a normal radiographic appearance. Infrabony defects may not be identified on the radiograph if the defects are relatively small. Radiography of a gutta-percha point inserted into the pocket may be helpful to evaluate the extent of the defect.

Advanced Periodontal Lesions

Stage four disease is represented by deep pockets, tooth mobility, gingival bleeding, and purulent discharge. Bone loss is extensive (Fig. 5.63).

Furcation exposure results from bone loss at the root junction of multirooted teeth (Figs. 5.64 and 5.65). Furcation exposure indicates advanced periodontal disease. It is sometimes difficult to determine radiographically whether the interadicular space is involved unless there is a radiolucent area in the region of the furcation. Advanced furcation exposures where both cortical plates are compromised are easily recognized on radiographs.

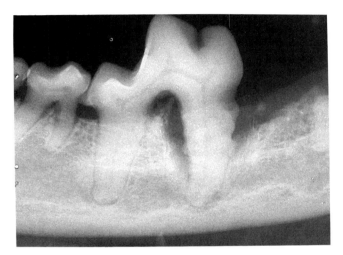

Fig. 5.61. Vertical bone loss affecting distal root of mandibular first molar.

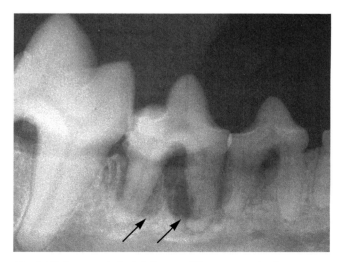

Fig. 5.62. Severe periodontal disease with accompanying bone loss (arrows).

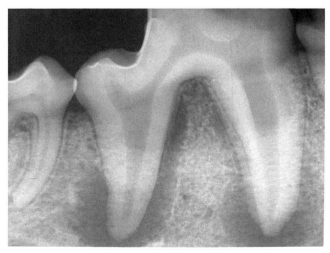

Fig. 5.63. Endoperio lesion. Note periapical (white arrow) *and periodontal bone loss* (black arrow).

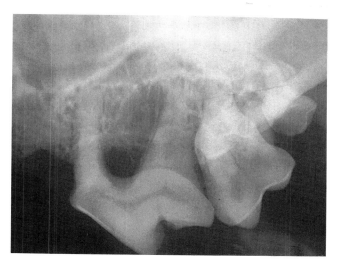

Fig. 5.64. Radiographic appearance of normal alveolar bone in furcation of maxillary fourth premolar.

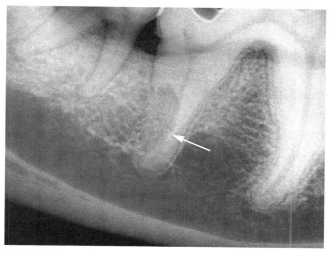

Fig. 5.66. External resorptive lesion on root of mandibular first molar (arrow).

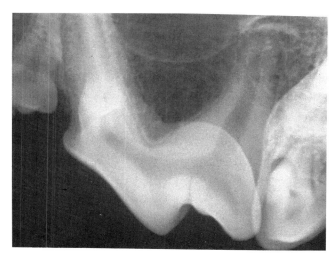

Fig. 5.65. Note bone loss at furcation secondary to grade three periodontal disease.

Alveolar dehiscence exists when alveolar cortical bone is resorbed along the entire length of the root. Radiographically, there will be radiolucency surrounding the affected root.

Radiology of Endodontic Disease

The 40 percent rule is *40 percent of the bone has to be destroyed before you can see periapical lucency on a radiograph.* When examining radiographs, just because you may not see lesions does not mean they are not present.

External resorption begins on the surface of the tooth (Fig. 5.66). The resorption may result from periapical inflammation, excessive occlusal forces, or unknown stimuli.

Internal resorption arises from within the pulp (Fig. 5.67). The cause is unknown, but trauma is believed to be a contributing factor. Often, it is difficult to determine if the lesion is due to internal or external resorption. If you see a normal appearing root canal through the resorption, then the lesion is external in origin.

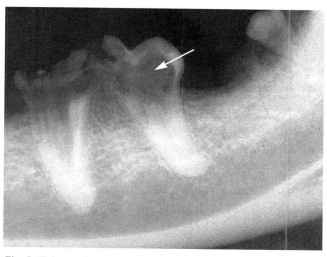

Fig. 5.67. Internal resorption (arrow).

Periapical abscesses usually appear as a slight thickening of the apical periodontal ligament with minimal alveolar bone resorption. Most cases do not reveal extensive bone loss due to the short time period between pulp death and the formation of the periapical abscess.

A chronic purulent periapical abscess appears radiographically as a homogenous radiolucency at the root tip, with a dark halo in the periapical tissues (Fig. 5.68).

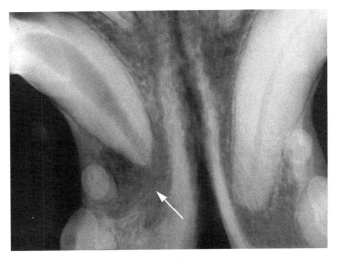

Fig. 5.68. Periapical abscess (arrow).

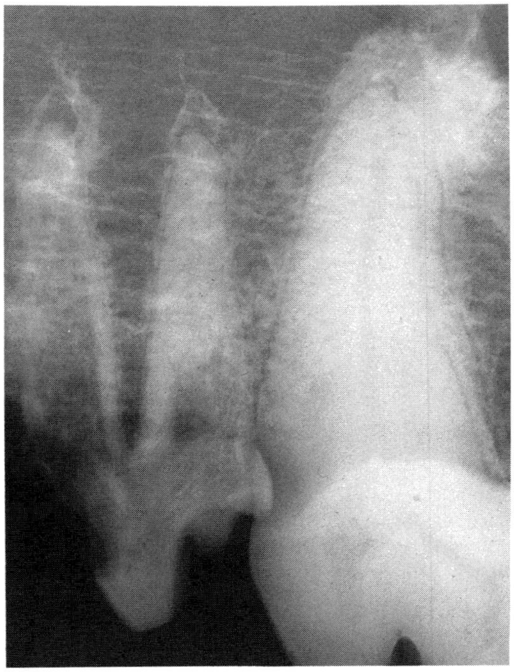

A **dental granuloma** appears as a radiolucent lesion with a circumscribed outline revealing a wall of compact cancellous bone. The apex of the tooth projects into the lesion.

A **radicular cyst** is a fluid-filled sac at the root apex of a nonvital tooth. Radiographically, it will appear as a rounded, circumscribed, radiolucency bounded by an unbroken line of sclerotic bone (Fig. 5.69).

Condensing osteitis occurs in response to low-grade infection. It appears as a small radiodense area around the root apex of a tooth circumscribed by a large area of denser bone (Fig. 5.70). The tooth is nonvital.

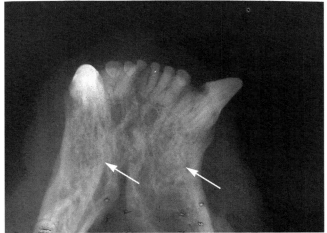

Fig. 5.70. Condensing osteitis at mesial apex of mandibular first molar (arrow).

Miscellaneous Conditions Diagnosed with the Aid of Radiography

Ankylosis—A tooth is ankylosed when there is union between the tooth root and alveolar bone (Fig. 5.71). The union is cementum to bone. Causes of ankylosed teeth include traumatic injury, occlusal trauma, and periapical inflammation.

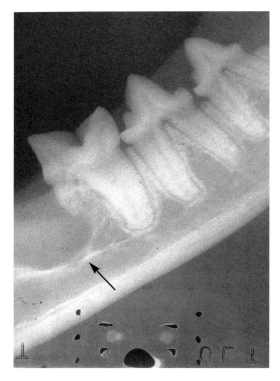

Fig. 5.69. Radicular cyst (arrow).

Fig. 5.71. Ankylosed tooth. Notice the absence of a clearly observable periodontal ligament (arrows).

Metabolic disease—Renal secondary hyperparathyroidism radiographically is portrayed as a generalized loss of bone support of all the teeth (Fig. 5.72).

Neoplasia—In radiographs, look for destruction of all tissues around the tooth (Fig. 5.73).

Foreign bodies—In all cases of oral swellings, or nasal discharge, radiographs must be taken (Fig. 5.74).

As you can see, radiology is a vital diagnostic tool for diagnosing dental pathology. Essential therapy decisions are based on radiographic findings.

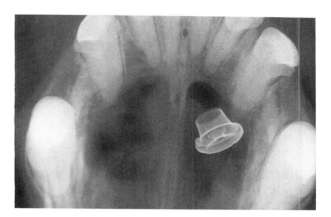

Fig. 5.74. Metallic foreign body in nasal cavity of dog with base narrow canines and one-year history of nasal discharge.

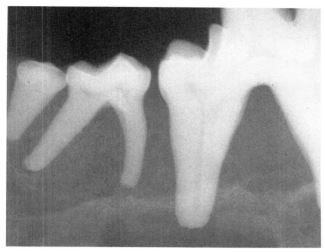

Fig. 5.72. Mandible from dog affected by renal secondary hyperparathyroidism. Note loss of alveolar bone.

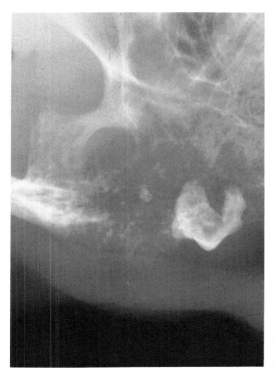

Fig. 5.73. Neoplasia— squamous cell carcinoma in a cat.

6. TWELVE STEPS OF THE PROFESSIONAL TEETH-CLEANING VISIT

No matter how trifling the matter on hand,
do it with a feeling that it demands the best that is
in you, and when done, look it over with a critical eye,
not sparing strict judgement of yourself.
—SIR WILLIAM OSLER

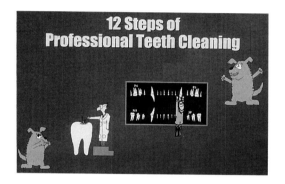

Fig. 6.1.

Prophy is an abbreviation of the word *prophylaxis*. In human dentistry, to prevent progression of dental disease, prophys include an examination, radiology when indicated, supra- and subgingival cleaning, as well as home care consultation. The dentist is usually presented with a relatively healthy mouth, and the hygienist cleans the patient's teeth and makes an appointment in three months to a year for another prophylaxis.

When used in the veterinary dentistry context, prophy is a catch-all term for teeth cleaning and most periodontal care. This needs to change. To call proper attention to what we are doing, we must more precisely describe teeth-cleaning procedures by identifying the extent of disease: for example, "teeth cleaning—grade one gingivitis," "teeth cleaning—grade two gingivitis," "teeth cleaning—established (grade three) periodontitis," and "teeth cleaning—advanced (grade four) periodontitis."

THE ROLE OF PLAQUE

Plaque forms a milky film on teeth and gums. As plaque accumulates in the sulcus under the gum line, the types of bacteria change, and bacterial by-products begin to destroy bone and tooth support. Control plaque, and you prevent periodontal disease.

Tartar, or calculus, is mineralized plaque. Tartar forms within days after calcium carbonate in saliva combines with plaque and hardens. This hard white or yellow substance sticks to teeth like cement and feels rough.

The oral cavities of dogs and cats are more alkaline than the human mouth, and plaque readily mineralizes with the higher animal salivary pH. This is a major reason periodontal destruction occurs five times more rapidly in dogs than in humans.

Smaller breeds are more predisposed to periodontal disease than large breeds.

- Small dogs have closer teeth, decreasing the effectiveness of the mouth's self-cleaning mechanisms.

- The smaller the pet, the thinner the bone that holds the tooth. Bacterial by-products destroy thinner bone faster than thicker bone.

- Bone is thinnest around the front teeth. This is why toy breeds commonly develop periodontal disease around the maxillary and mandibular incisors.

- Smaller dogs also live longer than larger breeds. The longer an animal lives, the more time periodontal disease has to cause damage.

- Many small dogs are open-mouth breathers. This dries out their mouths, decreasing saliva, which carries away germs.

THE FIRST 11 STEPS OF THE PROFESSIONAL TEETH-CLEANING VISIT

No other procedure performed on small animals does more to help them than periodic teeth cleaning and aftercare. The dental visit for cleaning must be performed in a methodical manner. All 12 steps are important and interlinked. When one step is not performed, the long-term benefit to the patient suffers.

1 Oral examination on the unanesthetized animal (Fig. 6.3). Begin with the face. Check for swellings and painful areas. Look at the eyes. Are they the same size? Is there swelling under one eye? Open and close the mouth to check for pain or crepitus in the temporomandibular joints. Grossly examine the teeth and gingiva for pathology. Try to examine each tooth rather than generally checking the mouth. If there is even only a small amount of tartar touching the gingiva, this is disease and needs immediate removal.

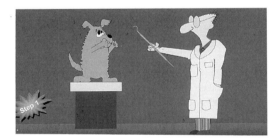

Fig. 6.2. Step 1. Oral examination on the unanesthetized animal.

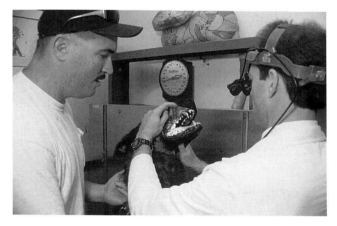

Fig. 6.3. First step of the teeth-cleaning visit: oral examination while dog is awake.

2 Oral examination under general anesthesia (Fig. 6.5). Examine individual teeth for mobility, fractures, malocclusion, and periodontal disease (probe for pocket depths after calculus is removed).

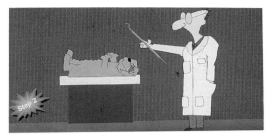

Fig. 6.4. Step 2. Oral examination under general anesthesia.

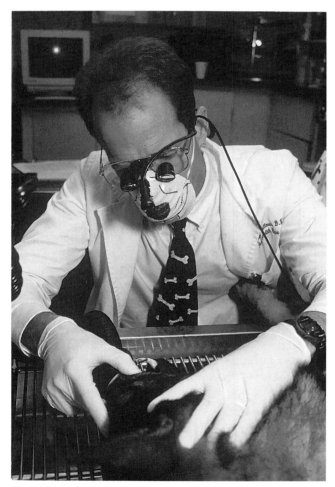

Fig. 6.5. Oral examination of dog under anesthesia.

3 Supragingival (above-the-gum-line) plaque and tartar removal using calculus-removing forceps, hand instruments, and power scaling equipment.

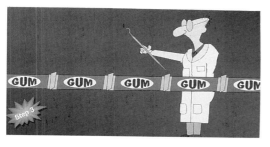

Fig. 6.6. Step 3. Supragingival (above-the-gum-line) plaque and tartar removal.

- Supragingival deposits are removed from buccal, lingual, and interproximal surfaces of the teeth.

- When used properly, the ultrasonic scaler removes plaque and tartar from the teeth (Fig. 6.7). Heat generated by an ultrasonic scaler can cause severe damage to the tooth and periodontal support. Ultrasonic units must be used only on crowns and exposed root surfaces unless specialized subgingival tips are used.

- The ability of an ultrasonic scaler to remove tartar and avoid potential damage depends on power settings, time of exposure, amount of pressure applied, and sharpness of the tip.

- Regardless of the type of power scaler, use a featherlight touch, keeping the water-cooled tip moving in a constant sweeping motion to avoid thermal injury. Use the side of the tip, not the point, to remove tartar.

4 Subgingival (below-the-gum-line) scaling, root planing, and curettage. Use curettes to remove subgingival deposits. Pockets greater than 5 mm require surgically exposing the root. The three parts of step four include

- **Root scaling:** Complete removal of plaque and calculus from the root surface. The goal is to disorganize and lavage bacteria living subgingivally. This creates a healthier environment for healing and reattachment. Curettes or slim ultrasonic tips are used (Figs. 6.9 and 6.10).

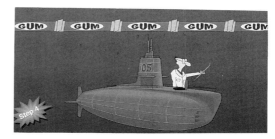

Fig. 6.8. Step 4. Subgingival (below-the-gum-line) scaling, root planing, and curettage.

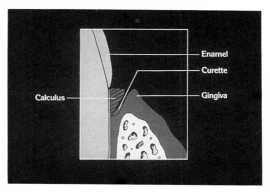

Fig. 6.9.

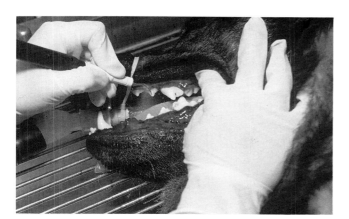

Fig. 6.7. Supragingival teeth cleaning with ultrasonic scaler.

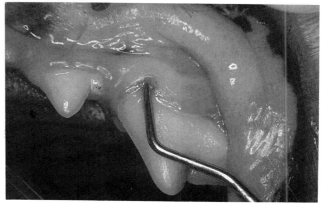

Fig. 6.10. Curette designed to be used subgingivally.

- **Root planing:** The smoothing of roughened root surfaces by debriding diseased cementum and removing embedded calculus to produce a clean, smooth surface free of endotoxin. Root planing is performed with a curette used in overlapping strokes. Crosshatch planing creates a smooth surface while maintaining root anatomy.

  Removal of all exposed cementum may *not* be helpful to periodontal health. Cementum contains chemicals that enhance reattachment of periodontal ligament. Bacteria do not penetrate into the cementum. Stripping cementum by root planing removes potential reattachment resources.

- **Subgingival curettage:** Removal of the gingival pocket's diseased soft tissue inner surface. The rationale for the procedure is to convert chronically inflamed ulcerated lesions in the soft tissue wall of a periodontal pocket into a clean surgical wound. This promotes healing and readaptation of tissue to the tooth surface.

  Subgingival curettage is done without direct visualization of the root surface. It is performed with a curette held in the reverse position. The blade is placed against the soft tissue for epithelial removal. The curette tip is used to remove remnants of the epithelial junction. This allows for optimal reattachment and reduction of the periodontal pocket.

5 **Polishing.** Regardless of how careful you are during the scaling/curettage phase of teeth cleaning, minor defects of the tooth surface occur. Polishing smooths out the defects and removes plaque missed during previous steps (Fig. 6.12). Pumice or polishing paste is used on a polishing cup for the procedure.

- When polishing, use firm pressure until the cup edge flares.

- Prevent overheating by relieving pressure slightly as you move the cup over each tooth.

- Avoid a bouncing stroke.

- Using continuous motion, keep the cup in contact with the tooth but do not hold the cup on one spot for more than a few seconds. Draw the cup over each tooth surface: begin at the gingival margin and move in a coronal direction.

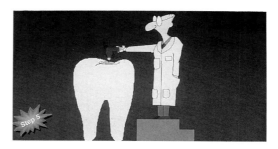

Fig. 6.11. Step 5. Polishing.

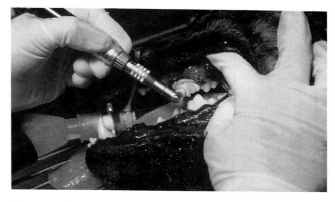

Fig. 6.12. Polishing after ultrasonic cleaning.

6 **Irrigation.** With irrigation, diseased tissue and plaque are removed from the pocket or sulcus (Fig. 6.14). Water spray and/or a 0.1–0.2 percent chlorhexidine gluconate solution are commonly used. Blunted 23-gauge needles are available for manual irrigation. Power irrigation is supplied on many delivery systems.

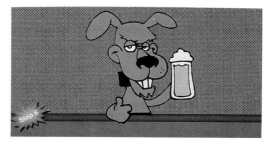

Fig. 6.13. Step 6. Irrigation.

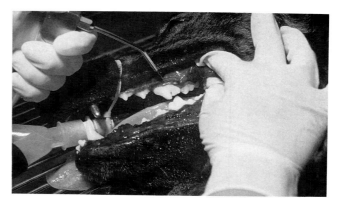

Fig. 6.14. Irrigation with air/water spray.

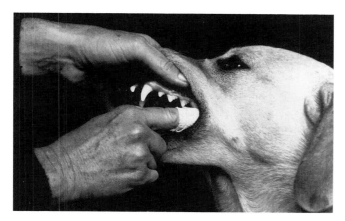

Fig. 6.26. Use of gauze sponge to clean teeth. This removes plaque above the gum line but cannot adequately clean below the gum line.

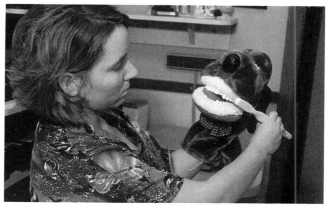

Fig. 6.27. Technician showing client how to use toothbrush on pet's teeth.

bond is enhanced when daily brushing is performed following instructions given at the animal hospital.

Staff members must be knowledgeable about tooth-brushing techniques in order to review the procedures with clients. Plastic models or a demonstrator animal can be used for training. Nothing beats hands-on instruction.

Clients often ask, "doesn't hard food keep teeth clean?" Some believe when their dogs or cats chew on hard food or biscuits that mineral deposits are broken down and the teeth stay clean. This is not true. Animals on soft diets accumulate plaque more readily than those on dry foods, but the only way to keep teeth clean above and below the gum line is by daily brushing.

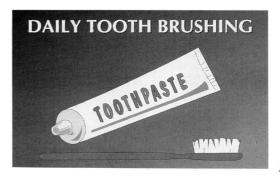

Fig. 6.28.

How to Teach the Client to Brush the Pet's Teeth

Brushing instructions must be more than telling your client it would be a good idea to brush the pet's teeth, then selling a toothbrush. The client needs to be shown how to properly use the toothbrush and toothpaste, and then he or she should be asked to perform the procedure in front of you (Fig. 6.27).

How to Get the Pet to Accept Toothbrushing

The proper technique for brushing teeth is applying the bristles at a 45-degree angle to the gingiva. Use small circular motions around the outside of the teeth and be sure to get the bristles under the gum line (Fig. 6.29). It is not as important to brush the inside of the teeth because dogs and cats do not have as much tartar on the palatal or lingual sides of their teeth as people do.

The most important area to keep clean is the sulcus under the free gingival margin. It is the plaque and tar

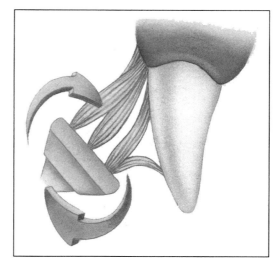

Fig. 6.29. Proper toothbrush bristle position.

tar underneath the gum line that is removed by daily home care. Adding products such as Oxyfresh to the drinking water or rubbing the teeth with dentifrice-impregnated pads may help in home care, but the client must understand that periodontal disease begins in the gingival sulcus. Home care is most effective when the dentifrice is brushed below the gum line. Instruct the client

- To start with a healthy, pain-free mouth. Untreated problems can cause a sore mouth and a noncompliant patient. Dental pathology must be cared for before the client is instructed to brush the pet's teeth.

- To choose a proper toothbrush and toothpaste. Toothbrushes have bristles that reach under the gum line and clean the space that surrounds each tooth. Plaque accumulates in this space. Devices such as gauze pads, sponge swabs, or cotton swabs remove plaque above the gum line but cannot adequately clean this space below the gum line.

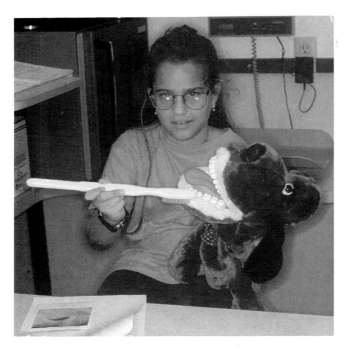

Fig. 6.30. Young helper showing client how to use toothbrush on pet's teeth.

The size of the toothbrush chosen is important. There are specially made brushes to fit into the large mouths of long-muzzled dogs as well as small brushes for cats.

Each dog or cat must have its own brush. Sharing brushes may result in cross contamination of pathogens from one pet to another.

- To introduce the pet to the toothpaste and toothbrush gradually (Figs. 6.31 and 6.32)

- To repeat and reward

- To reassure the pet by talking to it when it is anxious about the brushing procedure. Then the client should try again. The client should expect progress, not perfection, and reward progress immediately with a treat or a play period after each cleaning session.

Tell clients to take their time. Each pet is different. Some will be trained in one week while others will take a month or more. The payoff is well worth the learning curve.

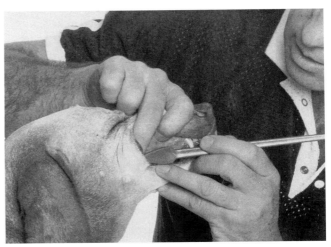

Fig. 6.31. Proper position for using dog toothbrush.

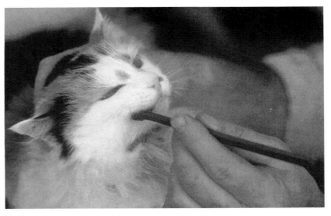

Fig. 6.32. How to hold a cat for toothbrushing.

Teeth-Cleaning Products

Human toothbrushes are usually too large and firm for animals. Specially engineered veterinary toothbrushes work well. Advantages of using a toothbrush for home care include

- It has soft bristles that can reach subgingivally, cleaning the sulcus.

- It can be used to apply toothpaste or medication below the gum line.
- It will mechanically remove plaque.

Disadvantages:

- It may be bulky and difficult for the owner to use.
- It can traumatize the gingiva.
- It may cause pain to the small animal.
- It may harbor bacteria in the bristles.

VRX Pharmaceuticals (Harbor City, California) produces five types of toothbrushes designed specifically for use in small animals (Figs. 6.33–6.35).

- The **puppy toothbrush** (*A*) has a small head to accommodate a smaller mouth. Bristles are ultrasoft for gentle application.

- The **dual-ended toothbrush** (*B*) has head sizes to adapt to both small and large tooth surfaces. The long handle and reverse-angle heads help usage.

- The **feline toothbrush** (*C*) allows a stroking or swabbing motion in small cats' mouths. Bristles are soft to ensure a gentle application.

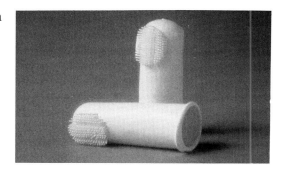

Fig. 6.34. Finger toothbrush.

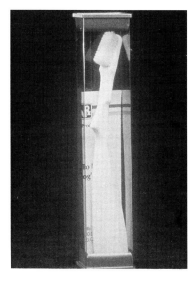

Fig. 6.35. Adult canine toothbrush.

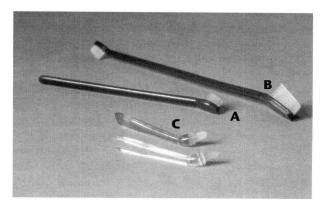

Fig. 6.33. Small animal toothbrushes available from VRX Pharmaceuticals. A = puppy toothbrush, B = dual-ended toothbrush, C = feline toothbrush.

- The **finger toothbrush** is popular for beginners (Fig. 6.34). It fits on the end of the pet owner's index finger, which reduces the resistance of both pet and owner. The brush will remove plaque from the tooth surface, and it can be cleaned in a dishwasher.
  Unfortunately, the finger brush's working end does not extend subgingivally to remove plaque. This brush must be regarded as a tool to get the pet used to brushing so that a bristled brush may be introduced into daily home care.

- The **canine toothbrush** has a sturdy, molded handle for a secure grip (Fig. 6.35). The reverse-angle, curved head provides greater control and visibility while brushing.

Nylabone Products produces a 2-Brush system to brush both sides of the teeth at the same time. The toothbrush also comes with toothpaste incorporated into the bristles.

Hand scalers and curettes must not be used by clients, no matter what degree of professional training they have. Hand scaling can easily cause trauma to the gingiva in an unanesthetized dog or cat.

Dentifrices (dental cleansers) are aids to cleaning and polishing tooth surfaces. Human toothpaste must not be used on dogs and cats because it contains detergents that should not be swallowed.

Dentifrices are marketed in many forms:

- Powders, which are not used routinely because they can irritate the eyes and be accidentally inhaled. Baking soda, while mildly abrasive, tastes bitter and, due to the sodium content, may not be appropriate for dogs and cats with heart problems.

• Liquids, which are delivered as sprays to the teeth

• Gels and pastes, which are effective because they adhere to the toothbrush and tooth surface

— DVM/Doggy Dent Toothpaste contains a flavoring that encourages patient acceptance of the brushing process.
— VRX Pharmaceuticals' lactoperoxidase system enzyme-enhanced products come in meat- or malt-flavored pastes, which also have antibacterial properties that decrease plaque.
— CET FORTE Toothpaste (VRX Pharmaceuticals) has an extrastrength enzyme system with increased abrasiveness (Fig. 6.36). It is made for dog owners who do not brush their pets' teeth daily.

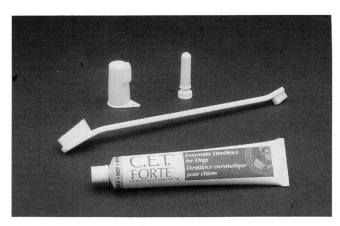

Fig. 6.36. CET FORTE Toothpaste.

TEETH-CLEANING PRODUCTS FOR DOGS AND CATS WITH PERIODONTAL DISEASE

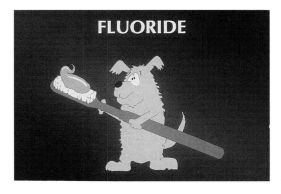

Fig. 6.37.

• **Fluoride** products

— Stannous fluoride preparations have advantages in helping to control periodontal disease because they reduce plaque and dental pain. A 0.4 percent strength should be used in patients with stage three or four periodontal disease. Use a blunted pe-

riodontal needle to infuse stannous fluoride into the pocket.

• Omni Gel (Dunhall Pharmaceuticals, Inc., Stafford, Texas)
• Gel Kam (Gel Kam International, Dallas, Texas)

— Sodium fluoride is commonly incorporated in human toothpastes. It is active at a pH of 3–4 and at this pH will replace calcium on the tooth with fluoride. Due to its acid content, it is not a good product for home care.

• Flurafom (VRX Pharmaceuticals) is a foam used after professional teeth cleaning, while the animal is under anesthesia.

— Fluoride-containing pet toothpastes

• CET Poultry (VRX Pharmaceuticals)

• **Maxiguard** (Addison Biological Laboratory, Inc.) contains vitamin C and zinc gluconate, which may promote healing of ulcerated tissue by stimulating collagen formation.

• **Chlorhexidine** is the most effective product for inhibiting plaque formation in humans. Chlorhexidine produces bacteriostatic and bactericidal effects against bacteria, fungi, and some viruses. Once absorbed, it continues to be effective for up to 24 hours.

In humans, to be maximally effective, chlorhexidine is swished in the mouth for one minute twice daily. The contact time of application is important for chlorhexidine to bind to the tooth and gingival sulcus.

One-minute oral rinsing is difficult to accomplish in animals. Chlorhexidine can be applied with a gauze sponge or cotton-tipped applicator, as a spray, or with a finger brush.

For animals, chlorhexidine is available as

— CHX Guard Solution (VRX Pharmaceuticals), composed of 0.12 percent chlorhexidine gluconate plus zinc gluconate (Fig. 6.38). This solution may promote healing of ulcerated tissue.
— CHX Gel (VRX Pharmaceuticals), containing 0.12 percent chlorhexidine gluconate (Fig. 6.38). The gel allows greater binding time and a pleasant taste.
— Nolvadent, composed of 0.1 percent chlorhexidine acetate
— Hexarinse (Virbac), containing 0.12 percent chlor-

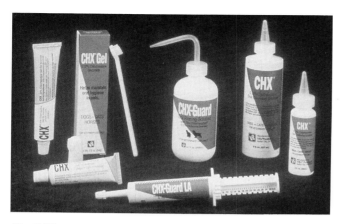

Fig. 6.38.

hexidine gluconate plus zinc

Chlorhexidine should not be used at the same time a fluoride product is used. Both may be inactivated by binding to each other. A 30-minute to one-hour wait is recommended between the use of a dentifrice containing fluoride and the use of a chlorhexidine rinse or gel.

- **Zinc** has been shown to enhance the antiplaque activity of chlorhexidine. Zinc reduces halitosis by inhibiting the production and release of volatile sulfur compounds. Zinc ascorbate also stimulates collagen production, which helps repair diseased tissue.

Zinc and chlorhexidine are available as CHX Guard Solution and Gel (VRX Pharmaceuticals) (Fig. 6.38) and as Hexarinse (Virbac). Zinc and vitamin C are available as Maxiguard (Addison Biological Laboratory, Inc.).

Chew Toys, Special Foods, and Dental Devices

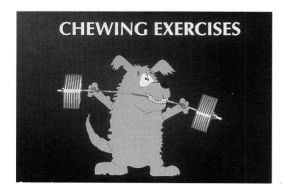

Fig. 6.39.

Often products claim to help keep small animals' mouths healthy. Unfortunately, many clients believe that giving their animals chew toys, without checking the toys' effectiveness, fulfills their responsibility for home care. The truth is that no chew toy really cleans plaque and tartar under the gum line, where disease occurs. Some products may even be dangerous. Chew toys do not take the place of daily brushing.

Some toys can even cause damage to a dog or cat. Beware of any toy with pieces that can break off. If the dog or cat inhales these pieces, they can obstruct the airway. Swallowing the pieces can result in intestinal obstruction.

Use of all chew toys and dental devices must be monitored. A pet can abuse any dental device. If the product is too soft, an aggressive dog will break it apart and swallow the pieces. If the product is too hard, tooth fractures may occur. Even tennis balls can cause problems from abrasion.

Beware of devices that are as hard or harder than teeth (Fig. 6.40). These include chew toys made from heavy plastic. When dogs bite on such products, they may wear teeth abnormally, removing areas of enamel and dentin, or cause a fracture. The most common chew toy causing dental problems is the cow hoof, which often causes fracture of the maxillary fourth premolar as well as other teeth.

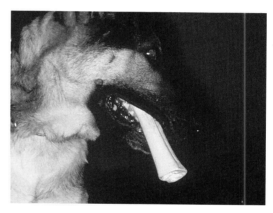

Fig. 6.40. Hard bones must not be given to dogs to chew.

The main benefit of dental devices and chew toys is chewing stimulation. Chewing removes some of the plaque and provides exercise to periodontal ligaments. Food manufacturers and toy makers have tried to create products to replace the need for toothbrushing. This has not been accomplished. At best, the products serve as plaque-controlling aids. Some examples of products available:

- Rawhide strips, such as CET Chews (VRX Pharmaceuticals), ChewEzee (Friskies Petcare, Glendale, California), and Roar-Hide (Nylabone Products), are effective for controlling plaque when combined with toothbrushing. Rawhide chews are usually safely chewed and swallowed. Unfortunately, some dogs are "gulpers," swallowing the rawhide without chewing and potentially causing gastrointestinal problems.

- Kong toys (Kong Company, Lakewood, Colorado)

- DentaBone (Chum Rask) by Pedigree (Waltham, Vernon, California) is an oral hygiene chew made from rice and milk protein.

- DenTreats (VRX Pharmaceuticals), used as a treat to accompany toothbrushing, contains zinc to decrease halitosis.

- Nylabone dental products can help control tartar; however, some dogs break off sections of the plastic, resulting in dental or gastrointestinal problems.

  — Chick-n-Cheez Chooz is an edible chew toy.
  — Nylon chewing devices include Dental Dinosaur, Hercules, Galileo, and Plaque Attacker. Nylabone Products advertises "dental tips" on these toys for teeth cleaning and gum massage.
  — Gumabones are more pliable than the nylon bones.
  — Rhino is a specially designed dog dental device made of rubber. A Nylabone Products advertisement calls attention to "pyramids to maximize dog's chewing enjoyment while cleaning the teeth and exercising the jaws."

- CET FORTE Chews for cats contain freeze-dried fish treated with an antibacterial enzyme system to provide abrasive cleansing action (Fig. 6.41). The coarse texture of the processed fish helps remove plaque and food debris.

Diets That Promote Clean Teeth

Foods are marketed that help control tartar and gingivitis. These diets can be used proactively (1) to help prevent gingivitis or (2) once periodontal disease has occurred and been treated. Feeding a specialized tartar control diet does not take the place of daily toothbrushing. For clients that feed the diets and brush their pets' teeth, the interval between professional teeth-cleaning visits is usually months longer than before feeding the diet.

- Canine and feline T/D (Hill's Pet Nutrition, Inc.) is a kibble formulation with transverse fibers that squeegee tartar from the tooth surface (Figs. 6.42 and 6.43). When fed as the sole diet, T/D decreases supragingival plaque.

- Tartar Check (Heinz Pet Products) is a snack biscuit containing sodium hexametaphosphate to help control tartar.

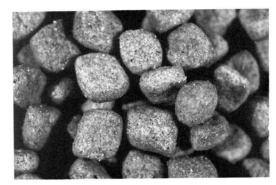

Fig. 6.42. Canine T/D.

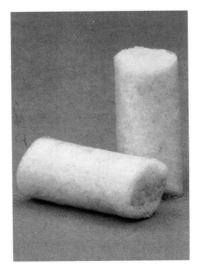

Fig. 6.41. CET FORTE Chews for cats (VRX Pharmaceuticals).

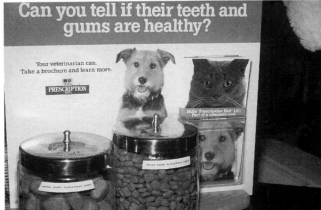

Fig. 6.43. T/D display.

How to Help Clients Practice Pet Dental Home Care

- Emphasize the benefits of brushing teeth: better breath, increased health, decreased pain, and hopefully a longer life.
- Keep the number of instructions for owners brief.
- Write down your recommendations.
- Use everyday language—limit confusing words.
- Be specific—include *what, when,* and *how* in your instructions.
- Show your clients how to brush their pets' teeth.
- Watch them perform the brushing.
- Ask for feedback: "So what do you think?"
- Use reminder cards and letters for interval-based professional rechecks.
- Follow up. Clients' compliance will be greatly increased when you show them you care.

How to Determine the Degree and Type of Home Care Products to Dispense

The degree and type of home care products used depend on the pet's stage of periodontal pathology.

- **Stages one and two:** Brush daily with a dentifrice.

- **Stage three** (periodontal disease has been established): Brush daily with a fluoride-containing toothpaste plus apply stannous fluoride gel twice weekly. Administer pulse therapy antibiotics.

- **Stage four** (advanced periodontal disease home care): Use zinc ascorbate spray three to four times daily plus 0.2 percent chlorhexidine spray twice daily. Or use CHX Guard Solution (VRX Pharmaceuticals), a combination of chlorhexidine gluconate and zinc. Administer pulse therapy antibiotics. At the end of two weeks, stannous fluoride gel used twice weekly can be substituted for the chlorhexidine spray.

THE TWELFTH STEP OF THE PROFESSIONAL TEETH-CLEANING VISIT

12 Follow-up progress visits. Follow-up visits are as essential as any of the preceding 11 steps. The time between oral exams is based on the degree of disease and the client's ability to provide home care. Some severe periodontal cases should be rechecked monthly, while pets that have been treated

for grade one gingivitis, and that have had their teeth brushed once or twice daily, can be rechecked every six months. In the practice's computer system, the interval for recheck can be linked to the degree of periodontal disease (i.e., if the client is charged for a grade three periodontal treatment, then a monthly reminder to check on home care is automatically generated).

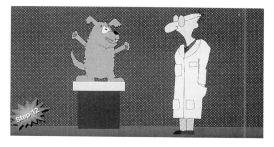

Fig. 6.44. Step 12. Follow-up progress visits.

OTHER TIPS FOR PROMOTING DENTAL CARE

- Have a dental health section in the merchandising area (Fig. 6.45). Include toothbrushes, toothpastes, chewies, and chew toys.

- Keep dental models in each exam room. Demonstrating oral pathology with the use of a model is easier than attempting to use a noncompliant pet.

- Use dental charts for every oral case to explain what was found in the oral examination, what was treated, and where the client needs to spend additional attention with home care.

- Training videos on home care are available from VRX Pharmaceuticals and Pharmacia & Upjohn Animal Health for client and staff instruction.

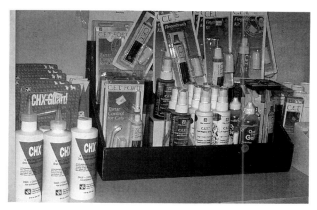

Fig. 6.45. Dental health merchandising area.

7. DECISIONS, DECISIONS, DECISIONS: Periodontal, Endodontic, Feline Oral, and Orthodontic Care

Every noble work is at first impossible.
—THOMAS CARLYLE

Once the dental examination is complete, and each tooth evaluated (visually, with probing, and through radiology if indicated), therapy is proposed to the client. Your clients are the owners of the dental team. It is up to them to hire or fire you. Their decision to accept or reject your recommendations is based on many factors, which in the end filter down to their pets' needs versus your wants. Your clients must be convinced that their pets need dental care in order to stay healthy. Just advising that their pets should have oral care is generally not enough. Describing the disease process, why care must be provided, and the sequelae if dental therapy is not performed will promote client acceptance.

The **treatment plan** is a carefully sequenced series of services designed to repair existing conditions and create a functional and maintainable environment. A sound treatment plan depends on thorough patient evaluation, dental expertise, and an accurate prognosis for each tooth.

Treatment planning is approached in phases. Planning for one procedure may be dependent on the success of another. The client's eagerness and the patient's ease of handling may also influence the planning process. For example, if a client's past home care efforts fail in reducing the amount of dental plaque in the animal's mouth, extensive periodontal procedures should not be suggested or performed. In such a case, extractions of teeth affected by marked periodontal disease would be the best approach.

While the veterinarian's long-range treatment goal may be idealistic, it is not necessary to immediately perform definitive treatment that will restore the mouth to the maximum degree of health and function. Urgent problems must be resolved before the veterinarian can focus on the goals he or she wishes to attain. This is especially true with periodontal disease. **Staging** the treatment plan over weeks to months works well. Initial care may consist of teeth cleaning, root planing, and extractions, followed by several weeks of antibiotics and home care, then reevaluation and flap surgery if still necessary.

Veterinarians must examine their own capabilities and appreciate their limitations when they determine the extent of treatment they are comfortable performing. Ignoring a fractured tooth with pulpal exposure is not good medicine. *Veterinarians must feel comfortable referring a patient having complex dental needs to a colleague with greater experience or expertise.*

Client education at the initial appointment is essential. Discussion must include

- How or why the condition developed
- Procedures necessary to treat the problem
- Prognosis
- What would happen if treatment was not performed
- Home care responsibilities
- What is necessary to prevent reoccurrence
- Fees related to present and future care for the problem

There are two types of treatment plans: an ideal plan and an optimal. The **ideal plan** is developed for situations where there are no constraints on the client's ability to accept the best therapy or on the practitioner's knowledge to perform said treatment or to refer. Examples of the ideal plan include guided tissue regeneration to save advanced periodontal disease–affected teeth and crown lengthening with metallic restoration after endodontics for subgingivally fractured teeth.

The **optimal plan** will adequately care for the patient's needs. The optimal plan should solve the problem even if it does not produce the ideal solution. Teeth affected with grades three and four periodontal disease would be extracted as well as fractured teeth with pulpal exposure if the optimal plan was chosen.

IMMEDIATE, INTERIM, AND MAINTENANCE CARE

The extent of a dog's or cat's disease dictates the treatment plan process required to achieve the maximum level of oral health. Some patients need only immediate treatment to care for a problem, while others will require immediate, interim, and maintenance care.

Immediate treatment is the initial care given for the client's complaint or the most pressing oral exam finding. The nature of the chief complaint and physical exam findings will dictate urgency of treatment. The goal of immediate treatment is to care for the most pressing problems, to prescribe treatment, and to schedule a reevaluation. An example of an immediate care treatment plan would be the extraction of grade four periodontal diseased teeth, gross calculus removal from the remaining teeth, deep scaling and polishing of teeth, and antibiotics.

Interim care is the second step. After a period of initial healing has taken place, the patient is examined. Additional therapy is performed if indicated.

Maintenance follow-up care is essential to long-term success. Probing, charting, and radiography are repeated every three to six months for advanced periodontal disease. Pulse therapy antibiotics may be indicated. These diagnostic procedures allow the veterinarian to evaluate the overall treatment plan, home care, and the patient's response to therapy.

Following are some common oral conditions and their care.

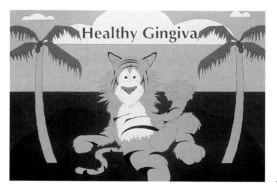

Fig. 7.1.

ORAL CONDITIONS REQUIRING PERIODONTAL CARE

Periodontal therapy involves removing calculus, detoxifying roots, providing surgery to access the roots, performing bone grafts, and motivating clients to carry out an effective oral hygiene program. In no other area of the body can a veterinarian make such a positive difference to long-term animal health.

The term *periodontium* is used to describe tissues that support the teeth, including

• The gums (gingiva)
• Periodontal ligament
• Alveolar bone
• Cementum

Teeth are supported in alveolar sockets by the periodontal ligaments, which attach from the alveolar bone to cementum covering the root. The periodontal ligament acts as a shock absorber for occlusal forces and an epithelial attachment to keep debris from entering deeper tissues.

The entire oral cavity is lined with mucosa. Keratinized surfaces of the mucosal lining (palate, tongue, and gingiva) are referred to as **masticatory mucosa** and the nonkeratinized surfaces are called the **alveolar mucosa**. The mucous membrane, which covers the alveolar process and makes contact with and attaches to the tooth, can be divided into two zones:

• **Keratinized tissue** is called the gingiva (Fig 7.2). The most coronal (toward the crown) aspect is referred to as the **free gingival margin (FGM)**. In a healthy dog the free gingival margin is 1–2 mm coronal to the **cemento-enamel junction (CEJ)**; in the cat, 0.5–1 mm. The junction of the gingiva with the alveolar mucosa is the **mucogingival junction (MGJ)** or **mucogingival line (MGL)**. Normal gingiva has a tough free margin with a sharp edge. The **free gingival margin** is held tightly around the tooth and is either coral pink or black pigmented. The **attached gingiva**, apical to the free margin, is also tough and normally tightly held to the underlying bone. Around the circumference of each tooth is a 0.5- to 2-mm **gingival sulcus**, where the sulcular epithelium of the gingiva contacts but does not attach to the tooth. This space between the gingiva and the tooth is also referred to as the gingival crevice.

• The **alveolar mucosa** is loosely attached nonkeratinized tissue located apical to the mucogingival junction. Alveolar mucosa is thin and less firmly bound to the underlying bone compared with attached gingiva.

Periodontal disease starts with the formation of plaque, a transparent adhesive fluid composed of mucin, sloughed epithelial cells, and gram-positive, aerobic cocci. Plaque starts forming within days after dental cleaning. Within a week, if plaque is not removed, mineral salts in the saliva precipitate on the plaque to form hard dental **calculus** (Fig. 7.3).

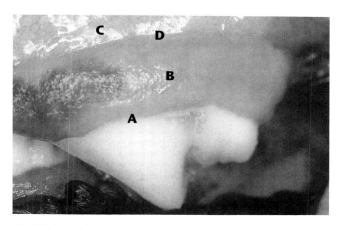

Fig. 7.2. Normal gingiva: (A) *free gingival margin,* (B) *attached gingiva,* (C) *alveolar mucosa,* (D) *mucogingival junction.*

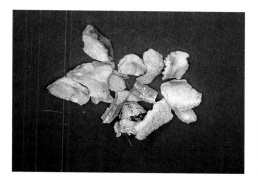

Fig. 7.3. Calculus removed from a dog's teeth.

Calculus is always covered with bacteria. The calculus plays a major role in maintaining and accelerating periodontal disease by keeping bacteria in close contact with the gingival tissue. Where calculus is present, gingival tissues become inflamed. If calculus is present in deep subgingival tissues, the potential for repair and new attachment without surgery is slim. *The therapeutic importance of removing calculus professionally and your client maintaining oral hygiene cannot be overemphasized.*

There is little difference between the bacteria supragingival (above-the-gum-line) and subgingival (below-the-gum-line) in healthy gingival sites. Initially, supragingival plaque bacteria are gram-positive, nonmotile, aerobic cocci. Once calculus forms, gingival tissue is irritated, changing the pH of the mouth and allowing pathogenic, gram-negative, anaerobic bacteria to survive subgingivally. By-products of these bacteria may resorb support structures, eventually causing tooth mobility and loss of teeth.

Periodontal disease is a multifactor infection.

- **Breed**—Small breeds are more prone to periodontal disease due to the closeness of their teeth and the thinness of bone around the incisors.

- **General health**—Those animals that have compromised health cannot fight periodontal pathogens as well. Animals with dermatological disease often chew on their hair coats, embedding hair under the gum line, which promotes periodontal disease.

- **Diet**—A soft food diet promotes and maintains periodontal disease.

- **Age**—Older pets are more prone to periodontal disease.

Local effects of chronic periodontal disease occur in the gingiva and bone. The destruction of bone is responsible for loss of teeth. Height of alveolar bone is normally maintained by an equilibrium between bone formation and bone resorption. When resorption exceeds formation, bone height is reduced. In periodontal disease, the equilibrium is altered so that bone resorption exceeds bone formation.

Periodontal pockets form where gingival attachment is lost. Supragingival tartar and calculus spread subgingivally into these pockets. **Gingival recession** occurs secondary to alveolar bone loss (Fig. 7.4). Recession is the exposure of the root surface by an apical shift in position of the gingiva. Recession may be visible, where the root is clinically observable, or hidden, where the root is covered by minimally adhered attached gingiva (Fig. 7.5). Hidden recession can be measured by inserting a probe to the level of epithelial attachment.

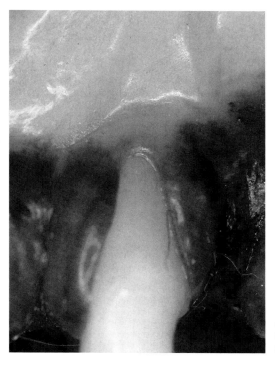

Fig. 7.4. Gingival recession.

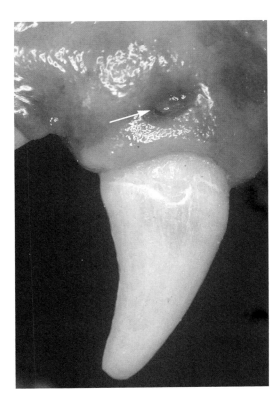

Fig. 7.5. Periodontal abscess (arrow).

The Periodontal Examination

Every professional teeth cleaning must include probing and charting. A periodontal probe is the single most important instrument used to evaluate periodontal health. A probe is marked in millimeter gradations and gently inserted in the space between the gingival margin and tooth. The probe stops where the gingiva attaches to the tooth or at the apex of the alveolus if the attachment is gone. Probing depths are measured from the base of the pocket to the margin of the free gingiva. Normal depths for dogs are 2 mm or less; for cats, 1 mm or less. Each tooth is probed on a minimum of four sides. Abnormal probing depths of all teeth are noted on the dental record.

Probing depth (pocket depth) is the distance from free gingival margin to the most apical point that a periodontal probe reaches when it is gently inserted into the gingival crevice.

Normally, the attached gingiva's coronal margin is within 1 mm of the CEJ in both the dog and cat. When gingival recession exists, **attachment loss** is a more accurate measure of periodontal disease than pocket depth is. Attachment loss levels are measured from the CEJ to the apical extent of the pocket. Pockets that result from attachment loss are called **periodontal pockets**. The periodontal pocket is a pathologically deep-ened gingival sulcus. Diagnosing periodontal disease and assessing response to treatment are based on this measurement. The measurement of pocket depth and attachment loss is the backbone of the periodontal examination.

Examination of the sulcular epithelium is important. By gently inserting the periodontal probe just apical to the free gingival margin and tracing the gingival crevice from mesial to distal, you can make a rapid determination of sulcular tissue health. If the lining is intact and healthy, there will be no bleeding. If there is disease, bleeding may occur.

When the tip of a probe extends into the periodontal pocket coronal to the supporting bone, a **suprabony pocket** exists. If the base of the pocket is apical to the supporting bone, an **infrabony pocket** exists (Fig. 7.6). Infrabony pockets are classified by the number of walls remaining around the tooth.

- **Three-wall defect**—There are three walls of bone surrounding the tooth. This pocket carries the best prognosis.

- **Two-wall defect**—Two walls of bone remain.

- **One-wall defect**—Only one wall of bone remains. This pocket carries a poor prognosis.

- **Cup** or **circumferential defect (four-wall)**—The defect completely surrounds the tooth.

When periodontal disease is not treated, subgingival anaerobic bacteria can continue to reproduce, creating deeper periodontal pockets through bone destruction. Eventually, this progression can cause tooth mobility and loss. The dog's or cat's general health may also be affected by the bacteria's extension into the kidney, heart, and liver.

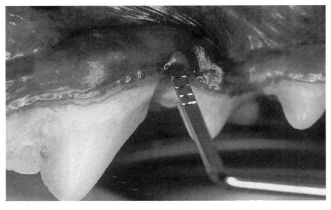

Fig. 7.6. Periodontal probe inserted in an infrabony pocket.

Gingivitis or Periodontitis?

There is a difference between gingivitis and periodontitis. **Gingivitis** is an inflammatory process affecting the soft tissue. This process does not clinically extend into the alveolar bone, periodontal ligament, or cementum. **Periodontitis** is inflammation involving the alveolar bone, periodontal ligament, and cementum. All cases of periodontitis start with gingivitis.

There are four stages of periodontal disease clinically recognizable.

Grade one disease (stage one gingivitis) appears as gingival inflammation and redness at the free gingival margin. Halitosis may be present (Fig. 7.7).

Grade two disease (advanced gingivitis) appears as free gingival inflammation, edema, and bleeding upon probing. There is no bone loss or tooth mobility. Calculus is present above and below the gum line (Fig. 7.8).

Grade three disease (established periodontitis) appears as moderate loss of attachment (< 50 percent), which shows clinically as pocket formation. Slight tooth mobility may be present. There may be pustular discharge upon probing (Fig. 7.9).

Grade four disease (advanced periodontitis) appears as marked (> 50 percent) bone loss, tooth mobility, and gingival recession, and there is attachment loss of greater than 50 percent (Fig. 7.10).

Figures 7.11–7.14 depict the four stages of periodontal disease in a cat; figures 7.15–7.18 depict the stages in a dog.

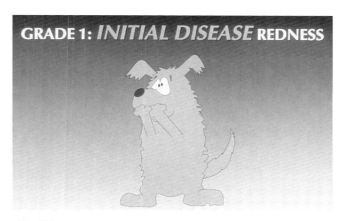

Fig. 7.7.

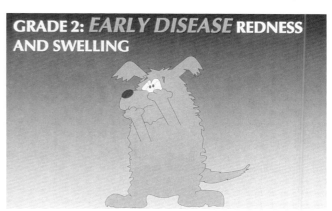

Fig. 7.8.

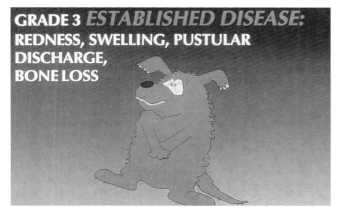

Fig. 7.9.

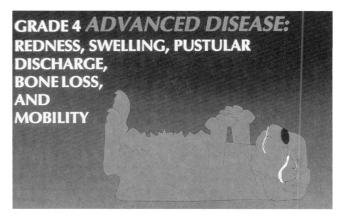

Fig. 7.10.

STAGES OF PERIODONTAL DISEASE IN A CAT

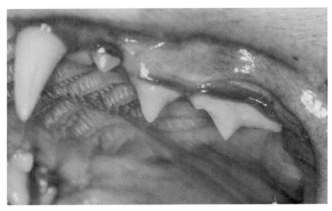

Fig. 7.11. *Feline maxillary premolars affected by grade one gingivitis. Note gingival inflammation.*

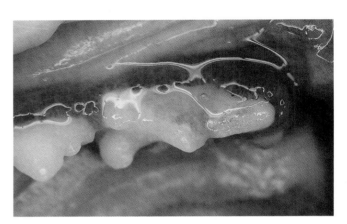

Fig. 7.12. *Feline maxillary fourth premolar affected by advanced gingivitis. Note inflammation and swelling.*

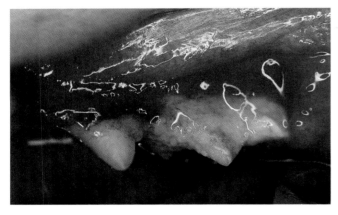

Fig. 7.13. *Feline established periodontal disease with bone loss and purulent discharge.*

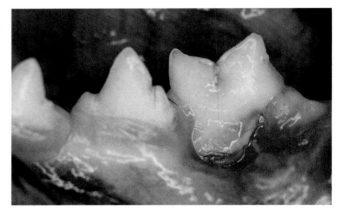

Fig. 7.14. *Feline mandibular molar affected by gingival recession secondary to advanced periodontal disease.*

STAGES OF PERIODONTAL DISEASE IN A DOG

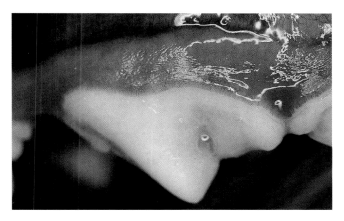

Fig. 7.15. Early gingivitis affecting the canine maxillary fourth premolar. Note gingival inflammation.

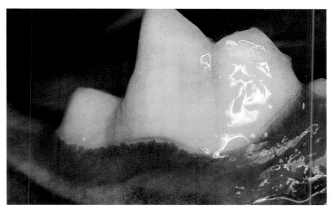

Fig. 7.16. Advanced gingivitis resulting in inflammation and swelling around the canine mandibular first molar.

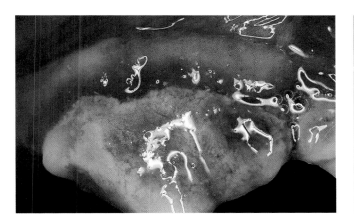

Fig. 7.17. Grade three periodontal disease around the canine maxillary fourth premolar.

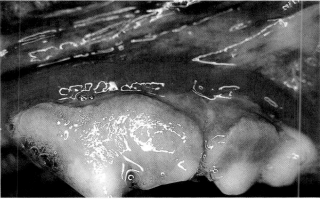

Fig. 7.18. Marked bone loss around the canine maxillary fourth premolar and first molar from grade four periodontal disease.

Periodontal Decisions

The goal of periodontal treatment is to free the tooth surface of calculus, plaque, debris, and diseased tissue in order to maintain healthy periodontal tissues. What criteria must the veterinarian evaluate when considering periodontal therapy?

- **The correct clients**—Most clients are committed to maintaining optimum pet health. Clients committed to pet health will, if given the opportunity, choose to save their pets' teeth. When determining if a client is a good candidate for accepting advanced periodontal pet care, the veterinarian must communicate that surgery does not permanently cure the animal's problem. The client's role in therapy includes

  —Daily brushing home care to remove plaque, which begins to colonize within 12 hours after a professional teeth cleaning
  —Returning for progress rechecks
  —Paying for dental care and aftercare

- **A cooperative, generally healthy patient**—The dog or cat must also be a willing partner. When a pet does not allow home care, the best dental surgeon and most caring owner cannot ensure long-term dental health.

- **The amount of bone remaining**—If less than 25 percent of bone remains supporting the tooth, advanced periodontal care will probably not provide long-term success.

Unless there is strong owner commitment and patient compliance, it is wiser to extract a tooth rather than allowing the pet to suffer.

Medical versus Surgical Therapy for Periodontal Disease

Once the clinician is convinced that he or she is working on the right patient and a salvageable tooth, the appropriate type of periodontal care is chosen. An ideal method allows

- Exposure of the root surface if the pocket is greater than 4 mm in the dog
- Preservation of the attached gingiva
- The gingiva to be resutured in a fashion that eliminates the periodontal pocket
- Reattachment of the gingiva to the root surface

Imagine a giant tooth sitting in a 10-ft garbage can containing mud and industrial waste. Continue to pretend it is your job to clean the tooth and you are supplied with equipment only 5 ft long. What happens? The top is cleaned, and the bottom is allowed to remain in the toxic waste until it eats through the can. How can you solve this problem? By opening the side of the can to clean waste out in order to save the tooth. This is the essence of periodontal surgery. Specific therapy decisions are based on probe depths, tooth mobility, and radiology findings.

GRADES ONE THROUGH FOUR PERIODONTAL DISEASE

Grades one and two gingival disease are treated nonsurgically. Once the teeth are cleaned and polished, fluoride is applied, and if home care is rigidly followed, the gingivitis clears up, and the gingiva returns to normal appearance and function.

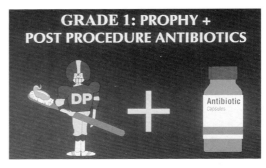

Fig. 7.19.

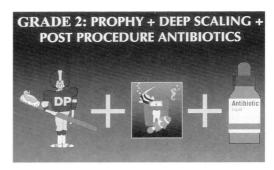

Fig. 7.20.

Grade three periodontal disease may require surgical care based on the amount of attachment loss. Once grade three occurs, there is permanent bone loss.

In the dog with pocket depths of 3–4 mm, and cat with depths of 2–3 mm, the subgingival area is cleaned with a curette. Ultrasonic scalers with specialized periodontal tips remove calculus and plaque and help return pockets to health.

Scaling, root planing, and curettage can be effective as definitive treatment techniques in periodontal disease where there is pocketing of 4–5 mm in the dog and

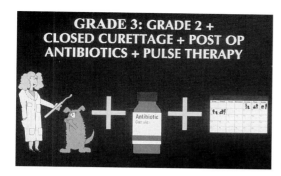

Fig. 7.21.

3–4 mm in the cat. The combination of tissue shrinkage, connective tissue remodeling, and gain of soft tissue attachment makes these procedures viable options.

- **Scaling**—Scaling removes calculus, heavy stains, and debris from the crown and gingival margin. The process removes primary irritants to the gingival tissues and reduces inflammation. Ultrasonic, subsonic, and hand instruments may be used.

- **Root planing**—Root surfaces exposed to periodontal disease are covered with bacterial plaque and endotoxin. When calculus is removed from the root surface, cementum is often left rough. Root planing, or shaving the root surface with a curette, will smooth these roughened surfaces (Figs. 7.22 and 7.23). Smooth surfaces are easier to keep clean than rough ones. The smooth surface will also adapt more easily to the cleaned pocket, reducing pocket depth. Aggressive root planing should be avoided because the cementum is helpful in the reattachment process.

- **Subgingival curettage**—Subgingival curettage involves removing the lining of the periodontal pocket as well as damaged tissue. Subgingival curettage is performed with the curette after plaque and calculus are removed.

- **Perioceutic treatment** (Heska)—Doxycycline gel injected into cleaned pockets greater than 4 mm in the dog will incorporate into the diseased tissues (Figs. 7.24 and 7.25). The gel physically remains for up to two weeks after application.

For pocket depths greater than 5 mm in dogs and 4 mm in cats, surgery is indicated. Pockets are the result of a disease process, rather than a disease. Mere pocket elimination by surgical methods will not cure periodontal disease. The rationale for surgical therapy is that it will improve access to calculus and facilitate calculus debridement and pocket elimination. The importance of maintenance therapy as opposed to one-stop

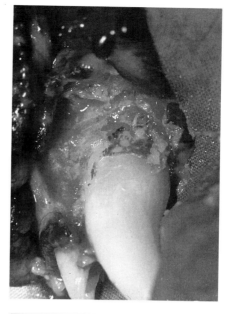

Fig. 7.22. Open flap exposing subgingival calculus.

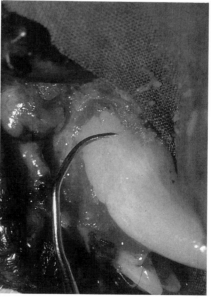

Fig. 7.23. Root planing on exposed root surface.

active therapy must be appreciated and conveyed to your clients.

Grade four periodontal disease requires surgical care: either extraction or periodontal surgery to gain exposure for root therapy and pocket elimination. The type of surgery depends on pocket classification as determined by probing and dental radiographs.

- A **suprabony pocket** exists where the epithelial attachment is coronal to the bony defect and is associated with horizontal bone loss. Suprabony lesions are often treated with mucoperiosteal flaps and osteoplasty.

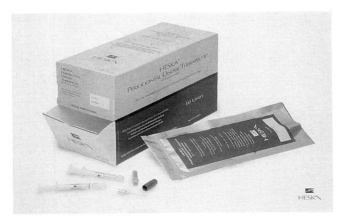

Fig. 7.24. Heska's perioceutic.

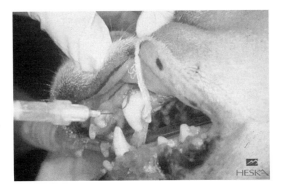

Fig. 7.25. Perioceutic applied to cleaned 5-mm pocket.

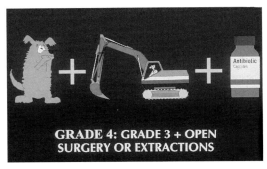

GRADE 4: GRADE 3 + OPEN SURGERY OR EXTRACTIONS

Fig. 7.26.

- If the epithelial attachment on the root surface is below the crest of bone, then it is an **infrabony pocket**, which is associated with vertical bone loss. Infrabony pockets are classified according to the number of bony walls left in the defect (one-, two- or three-wall lesions). Infrabony pockets can be treated with mucoperiosteal flaps, osteoplasty, bone grafts, and repositioned flaps.

Flap surgery is the most appropriate procedure to expose pathology of grade four periodontal disease and to render care. There are four commonly used methods in small animal dentistry: open flap curettage, apical repositioned flap, reverse bevel flap, and canine palatal flap.

Open flap curettage provides pocket reduction and encourages reattachment by allowing access to subgingival calculus and pocket epithelium. Open flap curettage is indicated in areas with pocket depths greater than 5 mm in the dog and 4 mm in the cat and where a better view is needed. This flap, which is not reflected past the crestal bone, gives the clinician access to infrabony defects and root surfaces. Under direct vision, the defects can be carefully curetted, and the root surfaces planed.

- Incisions of 360 degrees are made into the pockets with the blade tip angled toward the tooth.

- Two interdental incisions are made to expose the tooth root. The incisions are not made past the mucogingival line.

- A periosteal elevator is used to elevate the flap and expose the tooth's root surface for cleaning and root planing.

- Interdental sutures are placed with 4-0 chromic gut on an atraumatic needle.

The **apical repositioned flap** procedure, as shown in Figures 7.27–7.30, is used where the clinician wants to decrease the height of the pocket in areas of alveolar bone loss. This procedure is of value when pockets are apical to the mucogingival junction. An apical repositioned flap is a surgical creation of gingival recession to eliminate the pocket. The main goal is to reposition the gingiva so it overlies the alveolar bone, with the margin extending 2 mm coronally. One- and two-wall infrabony defects are treated with the apical repositioned flap.

- The blade is inserted 360 degrees around the tooth to incise the epithelial attachment.

- Vertical interdental incisions apical to the mucogingival line are made 2–3 mm mesial and distal to the affected tooth.

- A periosteal elevator is used to reflect the gingiva and expose alveolar bone. Sharp projections of the alveolus are smoothed, necrotic debris is removed from the root surface, and the area is irrigated with chlorhexidine.

- The incised gingiva is resutured to the new height of the alveolar bone, thus reducing pocket depth.

The **reverse bevel flap** is indicated where there are inflamed and necrotic free gingival margins. Radi-

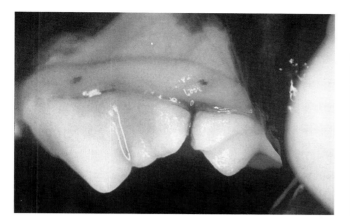

Fig. 7.27. Clinically observed grade four gingivitis.

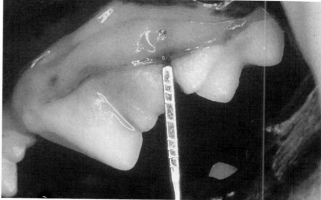

Fig. 7.28. Probe prior to insertion.

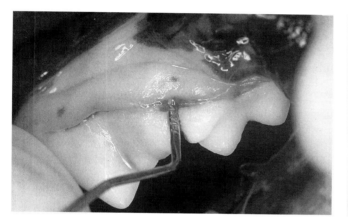

Fig. 7.29. Probe after inserting 9 mm into pocket.

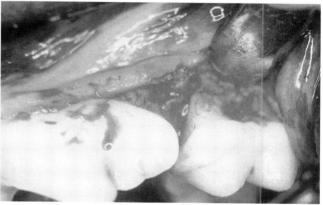

Fig. 7.30. Flap surgery exposing bone loss over mesial buccal root of maxillary first molar. An apical repositioned flap is performed to eliminate the pocket.

ographically, these areas may show as vertical infrabony defects. A portion of the diseased pocket epithelium is removed, providing access for root planing. Care must be taken to make sure that enough attached gingiva remains after the procedure. Single-walled defects repaired with bone grafts are best accessed via the reverse bevel flap.

- The initial incision is made parallel to the tooth between diseased and healthy appearing attached gingiva.

- At least 0.5 to 1 mm of attached gingiva is left as a collar around the affected tooth.

- The gingival collar is removed with a sharp curette, the root planed, the alveolar defects repaired, and the opposing edges of the "healthy" attached gingiva resutured.

The **canine palatal flap** is indicated where there are greater than 5-mm pockets on the palatal surface of the

canine teeth. If there is an oronasal fistula, as evidenced by sneezing or nasal discharge, and the probe enters the nasal cavity upon probing the palatal surface, then this procedure is not indicated, and extraction followed by single- or double-layered flap surgical closure of the defect is preferable.

- Four- to 8-mm incisions are made to the bone at a 20-degree angle palatally from the affected tooth.

- A periosteal elevator is used to expose the root for cleaning with hand instruments and the alveolus for application of various bone-filling materials in order to decrease the defect space and promote osseous integration.

- The area is closed with absorbable suture, such as 4-0 chromic gut on an atraumatic needle.

These therapy recommendations take into account that the gingival margin is near the cervical line and that the roots are approximately 10–15 mm in length.

Variations of these conditions will affect decisions about surgery. For example, given similar pocket depths, gingival margin levels apical to the cervical line make the prognosis less favorable than gingival margin levels coronal to the cervical line. Other considerations for whether or not to recommend periodontal surgery:

- **Client effort in patient plaque control**—Clients who have poor success in removing plaque from their pets' teeth will have pets that gain little over the long-term from periodontal surgery.

- **Value of the tooth**—The maxillary fourth premolar and mandibular first molars are the most "important" teeth because they act as scissors to cut food into smaller pieces. Molars are important for grinding food. Incisors and the first and second premolars perform the least important functions.

- **Age**—Younger animals can expect many years of use from saved teeth and will benefit more from advanced periodontal surgery than will aged animals.

FURCATION INVASIONS

Furcation invasions occur secondary to periodontal disease. The furcation is that area between the roots of multirooted teeth, formed where the roots begin to separate at the floor of the trunk. Normally, this area is sealed from the oral environment by the gingival attachment. The area of bifurcation or trifurcation is denuded when periodontal disease causes bone loss. Left untreated and allowed to progress, furcation invasion can result in tooth loss. There are three clinical furcation invasion classifications based on the use of an explorer probe.

- **F1**—Explorer can just detect an entrance to the furcation.
- **F2**—Explorer can enter the furcation but does not exit to the other side.
- **F3**—Explorer enters and exits through the other side.

Radiographs are helpful in locating furcation invasions. Diminished radiodensity in the furcation area suggests invasions. The slightest radiographic change in the furcation area should be clinically investigated.

Treatment for furcation involvement depends on the degree of invasion, ability of the veterinarian, and ability of the client to provide home care. The principles of surgical versus medical therapy, discussed earlier, apply. With marked furcation invasion, flap exposure can be performed, and a bone graft is applied to the area of bone loss, or the flap is repositioned apically to remove the pocket. When one or more roots are also affected by marked bone loss, the tooth can be sectioned, and a vital pulpotomy or root canal therapy can be performed on the "healthy root(s)," resulting in the ability to save the least affected part of the tooth.

For attachment loss greater than 9 mm in the dog and 6 mm in the cat, the value of even the most heroic surgery diminishes. Radiology plays a key role in the decision-making process. The amount of bone supporting a tooth helps determine when periodontal surgery will help to save a tooth or if it would be best extracted. *Generally, when greater than 50 percent of the bone remains supporting a tooth, periodontal surgery together with a healthy patient and strict home care will result in a saved tooth.* With new periodontal bone-grafting materials, this percentage is changing, with surgery helping to save teeth with less than 50 percent bone support. When less than 25 percent of bone support remains, the prognosis is so poor that surgery is usually not considered.

Intraoral radiography supplies important information when deciding which tooth can benefit from surgery. Radiographs help to evaluate supportive bone mesial (rostral) and distal to the affected tooth.

GINGIVAL HYPERPLASIA

In cases of **gingival hyperplasia**, there is an overgrowth of gingival tissue. The gingivectomy procedure employs a scalpel or electrosurgical blade to incise exuberant gingival tissue at a 45-degree angle toward the crown. At one time a gingivectomy was the treatment of choice to eliminate pockets and allow exposure of the root surface for cleaning. Unfortunately, part of the attached gingiva was sacrificed in the gingivectomy procedure.

Currently, all efforts are made to save valuable attached gingiva. Other surgical procedures such apical repositioned flaps and bone grafts help preserve attached gingiva. Gingivectomies are only used in cases of gingival hyperplasia.

ORONASAL FISTULAS

Oronasal fistulas result from periodontal disease of the maxillary teeth (most commonly canines), resulting in communication between the oral and nasal cavities (Fig. 7.31). A periodontal probe placed at the palatal aspect of maxillary canines will extend to the nasal cavity.

Clinical signs may include sneezing and nasal discharge, which is sometimes blood tinged. Repair of the fistula begins with the extraction of the canine tooth. Closure of the remaining defect via a buccal sliding flap (single-flap technique), followed by at least a week of antibiotics and oral rinses, is usually curative. A **buccal sliding flap** is used for repairing smaller acute fistulas.

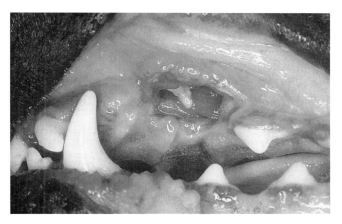

Fig. 7.31. Oronasal fistula.

Margins of the fistula are debrided circumferentially. A gingival flap is harvested and sutured to the edge of the fistula. Care is taken to avoid tension in the sutured flap.

A **double flap** is used when the fistula is chronic and/or large. Part of the palate is used to cover the defect. The palatal defect area is then covered with buccal mucosa to ensure a seal. Bone-grafting material can be placed within the defect before suturing.

MOBILE TEETH

Mobile teeth can be supported by adjacent nonmobile teeth with the help of a **periodontal splint** (Fig. 7.33). The splint cements one tooth to another. Strict home care is a must in order to save the splinted teeth.

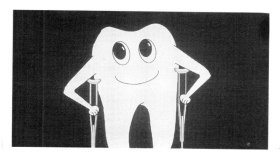

Fig. 7.32.

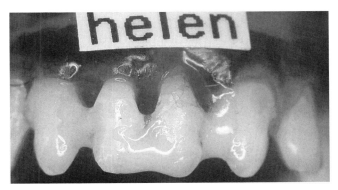

Fig. 7.33. Splinted incisors.

GUIDED TISSUE REGENERATION (GTR)

Bone and periodontal ligament can repopulate a periodontal disease–affected area with the help of **guided tissue regeneration**. One form of guided tissue regeneration is **bone grafting** (Figs. 7.35 and 7.36). Grafting prevents further bone loss and helps stabilize the tooth. Ideally, bone grafting restores normal bony architecture, rebuilds the periodontal ligament and soft tissue, and prevents periodontal pocket formation. Three-wall defects respond best to bone-grafting procedures.

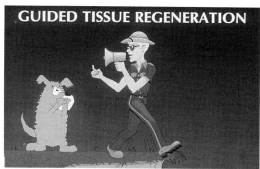

Fig. 7.34.

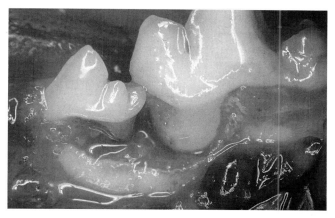

Fig. 7.35. Area of bone loss, exposed by flap.

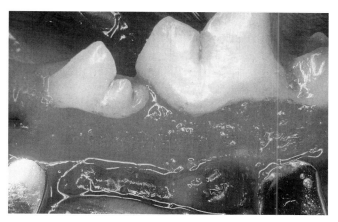

Fig. 7.36. Bone graft (Consil, by Nutrimax) placed over area of bone loss before flap closure.

Materials used for bone grafting include

- Synthetic bioactive bone (Consil by the Nurimax Company)
- Plaster of paris
- The animal's own bone
- Stored bone from cadavers

FRENULUM-RELATED PROBLEMS

The frenulum is a tough band of tissue connecting the inside surface of the lip to the mandibular gingiva near the first molar. A **mandibular frenectomy** is indicated when the frenulum causes gingival recession or pocket formation on the distal side of the mandibular canine teeth. By excising this attachment, food does not accumulate to irritate the pocket.

Postoperative Considerations for Periodontal Surgery

- Soften pet food for 72 hours after surgery. The client can easily do this by prewetting the animal's food for about 20 minutes before feeding.

- A 0.2 percent chlorhexidine solution is sent home with the owner to use twice daily for a week as an oral rinse to help wash away debris.

- Schedule a recheck appointment within three days.

- Intraoral dissolvable sutures will not need to be manually removed.

⟩Periodontal Care at a Glance

Problem	Appearance	Treatment
Grade one gingivitis	Plaque at gum line, inflammation. Halitosis is present	Oral exam before and after anesthesia, removal of supra- and subgingival calculas, irrigation, fluoride application, charting, home care instructions, follow-up visit scheduled in six months, one week of antibiotics
Grade two gingivitis	Calculus at gum line, inflammation and edema	Same as above plus intraoral radiology
Grade three periodontitis	Same as above plus probing attachment loss less than 50%	Same as above plus root planing. Possible perioceutic gel injection into cleaned pocket. Send home on pulse antibiotics.
Grade four periodontitis	Attachment loss greater than 50%, evidence of mobility, and/or gingival recession	Same as above plus curettage and surgery to save tooth through either flaps, guided tissue regeneration, or extraction
Furcation invasions	Gingival recession to exposure of void at area where the roots bifurcate or trifurcate	Flap surgery, guided tissue regeneration, hemisection where one or two roots cannot be saved based on loss of bone support, or extraction.
Oronasal fistula	Communication between the mouth and nasal cavity. Some animals will have a nasal discharge.	Extraction of the affected tooth plus closure of defect with single- or double-flap technique.
Severe gingival recession	Greater than 50 percent of root exposed	Intraoral radiographs to confirm findings, extraction or advanced periodontal care

ORAL CONDITIONS REQUIRING ENDODONTIC CARE

Care for the Fractured Tooth

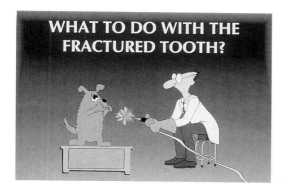

Fig. 7.37.

Endodontics is that branch of dentistry concerned with the anatomy, physiology, and pathology of the dental pulp and periapical tissues. Endodontics is a central and integral part of total patient care. The veterinary practitioner must be trained in endodontic evaluation and be prepared to perform endodontics, to extract the affected tooth, or to refer patients to practitioners who will perform therapy.

The term *root canal therapy* is feared by humans, who associate it with pain, difficulty, and expense. For these reasons, most veterinarians will not entertain the prospect of performing a root canal procedure. This decision is based on a lack of understanding. There are many important differences between root canal therapy in humans versus that in other animals:

- A majority of dog and cat root canals end in an apical delta without lateral canals. With humans, lateral canals are common and need to be sealed.

- Human root canal procedures are expected to last decades; animal procedures, years.

- Most human root canals are followed by crown restorations. Although crown restorations are preferable in pets, they are not essential for success.

- Human endodontic procedures require three to four visits; small animal root canal therapy is usually accomplished in one (two for crown restoration).

The veterinarian must not be afraid of learning how to perform endodontics. As with any new procedure, it is challenging at first and becomes easy after practice.

Root canal therapy has many advantages over extraction:

- The tooth is saved rather than the veterinarian resorting to "toothanasia."

- Root canal therapy is less invasive than surgical extraction, where removal of gingiva, bone, and tooth are involved.

- Less invasion causes less pain to the patient.

- In many cases, root canal therapy is faster than extraction, especially for a canine tooth.

Just because the animal doesn't appear to be in pain does not mean damage is not occurring. Often our patients do not "complain" to their owners or us about fractured teeth until lesions have progressed sometimes to the point of being untreatable. The days of observing and neglecting fractured teeth are over.

All teeth are susceptible to fracture; however, in the mature dog and cat, maxillary canines are most commonly broken, followed by the mandibular canines, the maxillary fourth premolars, and incisors. In the immature dog less than six months old, deciduous canine teeth commonly fracture.

How do small animals fracture their teeth? From chewing on cage doors, airplane crates, and chain-link fences. Also implicated are hard chew toys, ice cubes, and horse or cow hooves. Auto accidents, aggressive Schutzhund training, and dogfights can additionally lead to fractures.

Animals will experience pain when the tooth fractures. Eventually the pulp dies, and the pain decreases until an abscess forms. Animals show dental pain in many ways:

- Chewing on one side of the mouth
- Dropping food from the mouth when eating
- Drooling
- Pawing at the mouth
- Shying away when the face is petted
- Refusing to eat hard food
- Refusing to chew on toys

Endodontic Therapy Depending on Tooth Color

Often trauma does not result in loss of tooth structure. The tooth, however, is discolored, indicating pulpal hemorrhage. The ensuing inflammation (pulpitis) leads to increased pressure, causing tissue destruction

(Fig. 7.38). Bacteria can then move in through anachoresis (the process of bacteria lodging in an area of previously damaged tissue), causing lesions ranging from internal inflammation to an apical abscess. There are three color phases associated with pulpitis:

- **Pink** inflammation is sometimes reversible spontaneously or through immediate use of steroids and antibiotics. A reddish tint indicates red blood cells have leaked into the dentinal tubules from diseased odontoblasts. It is possible that the odontoblasts may recover. If the coronal tip of the tooth is the only part discolored, you may adopt a wait and see approach in which you take radiographs every six months. In a mature dog or cat, a better option is to perform root canal therapy on any discolored tooth.

- **Purple** indicates a dying tooth. The pulp is being strangled by the increased pressure. Root canal therapy is indicated.

- **Gray** or **brown** is the color of a dead tooth. Brown and gray teeth are also candidates for root canal therapy once radiographs indicate the tooth is salvageable.

Root canal therapy is indicated when you are faced with a discolored tooth. Waiting until radiographic changes appear means the animal will experience painful damage to the tooth and periapical support.

Endodontic Therapy Depending on the Parts of the Tooth Exposed

ENAMEL FRACTURE

Fractures involving the enamel only appear as chips in the enamel surface. The treatment of choice is to smooth any sharp edges with fine diamond burs and sanding disks in order to prevent trauma to the lips and tongue (Figs. 7.39 and 7.40). Intraoral radiographs must be taken to get baseline images of the root apex and to check for apical fractures. The tooth is reradiographed 6 and 12 months later for evidence of periapical pathology.

ENAMEL AND DENTIN FRACTURE

When the crown fracture involves enamel and dentin, bacteria have a direct pathway to the pulp through the dentinal tubules. This will be visually evident as a pink discoloration on the cut surface of the fracture. A method to diagnose pulpal exposure is to insert an explorer tip into the suspected exposed pulp. If the explorer tip does not penetrate, then pulp exposure is not present. Radiographs are taken for evaluation.

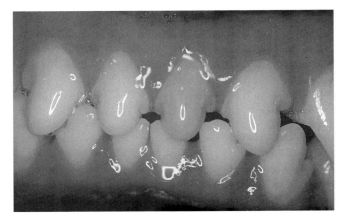

Fig. 7.38. Pulpitis. Notice gray-shaded left central incisor.

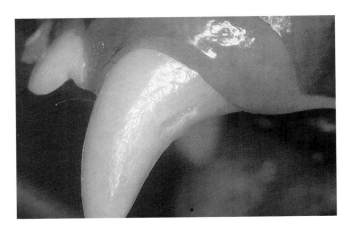

Fig. 7.39. Enamel fracture only.

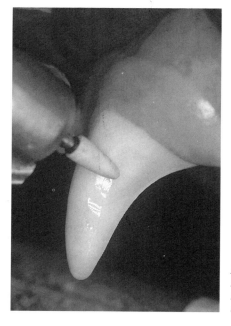

Fig. 7.40. White stone bur used to smooth out enamel defect.

Two therapy options to care for the tooth with enamel and dentin fractures are indirect and direct pulp capping.

- **Indirect pulp capping** covers exposed dentin with glass ionomer cement followed by crown restoration. For several years after the injury, follow-up radiographs are taken at six-month intervals to examine the pulp chamber for internal resorption and periapical pathology.

- **Direct pulp capping** involves removing dentin covering the pulp, placing calcium hydroxide or glass ionomer cement directly on the pulp, and then performing crown restoration (Figs. 7.41 and 7.42).

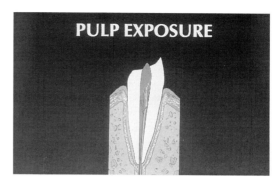

PULP EXPOSURE

Fig. 7.43.

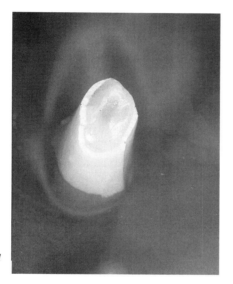

Fig. 7.41. Enamel and dentin fracture. The pulp is observable beneath fractured enamel and dentin.

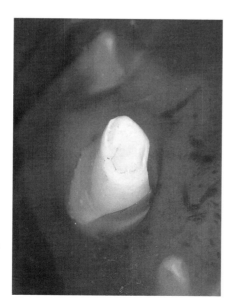

Fig. 7.42. Acrylic restoration of enamel and dentin fracture through direct pulp capping.

ENAMEL AND DENTIN FRACTURE WITH PULP EXPOSED

When the tooth fracture involves enamel and dentin, exposing the pulp, endodontic therapy is performed, or the tooth must be extracted. When the pulp is exposed, there is a direct communication between the oral bacterial environment and the bloodstream. An untreated exposed pulp leads to necrosis of tissue in the direction of the root apex. The process may be rapid, occurring in a month, or may be prolonged, with the tooth decaying for years.

With chronic inflammation of the pulp, dentin-resorbing cells may form. These cells cause resorption of the walls of the root canal, referred to as **internal resorption**.

Two variables that enter into the treatment decision-making process when pulp is exposed are the age of the fracture and the age of the patient.

Endodontic Therapy Depending on the Age of the Fracture

Immediately after pulpal exposure, and for up to two weeks, inflammation of the pulp exists less than 2 mm from the exposure site. When superficial necrosis occurs, healthy pulp tissue is found several millimeters deeper within the pulp. When the inflamed superficial layers of pulp are removed, the healthy pulp tissue will respond to vital pulp procedures. If the fracture is less than two weeks old, especially in a young patient, the vital pulpotomy may be performed. When the fracture is older than two weeks, or older than 48 hours in the mature patient, conventional or surgical endodontics is the treatment of choice.

VITAL PULPOTOMY

The advantages of vital pulpotomies:

- Ability to save a vital tooth
- Relatively easy to perform—few steps
- Usually takes 10-15 minutes to perform

The disadvantages of vital pulpotomies:

- May be sealing in infection that will cause problems
- Seal may leak in future
- Requires high-speed delivery system

Vital pulpotomies are indicated for

- Recent fractures (less than 48 hours) in a mature dog in an attempt to preserve the dental pulp
- Up to two weeks between the fracture and vital pulpotomy for younger animals (under 18 months old)
- Dogs or cats that undergo crown reduction procedures for orthodontic correction or for disarming

Vital pulpotomy procedure:

- A round or pear-shaped bur is used in a high-speed handpiece to remove approximately 5 mm (of a 10- to 15-mm-long tooth) from the coronal portion of the pulp.

- An inverted sterile paper point is applied gently to the pulp to control hemorrhage.

- Calcium hydroxide powder is applied with a retrograde amalgam carrier.

- When bleeding is controlled, 1 to 2 mm of self- or light-cured calcium hydroxide paste is applied on top of the powder.

- Glass ionomer cement may be used to cover the paste before the fracture site is restored.

- Acrylic bonding and/or metallic crowns are used for restoration.

- Postoperative antibiotics are given, and radiographs are taken at two-month intervals to evaluate the need for conventional endodontics.

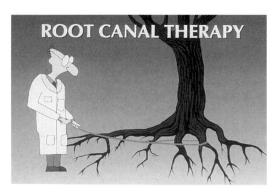

Fig. 7.44.

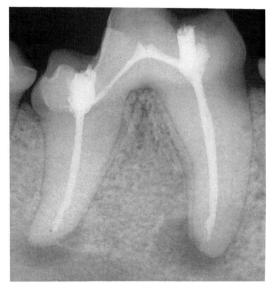

Fig. 7.45. Radiograph of tooth after root canal therapy.

CONVENTIONAL ENDODONTICS

In cases where the owners do not know when the fracture occurred, or if the fracture is older than two weeks in the young patient, or older than 48 hours in the mature patient, conventional or surgical root canal therapy (RCT) must be performed to remove affected pulp, to seal the apex, and to restore the crown. In cases where intraoral radiographs show marked periapical lysis, retrograde surgical endodontics or extraction is indicated.

Indications for Root Canal Therapy

- Fractured teeth with pulpal exposure more than two weeks in the young patient, or more than 48 hours in the mature patient, with fractured segments coronal to the free gingival margin

- Discolored teeth, which indicate pulpal death from trauma

- Periapical abscesses with or without fistula formation

Instrumentation for Root Canal Therapy

- "Hardware"

  — High-speed delivery system with assorted burs
  — Dental radiograph unit
  — Light cure for restoration of access hole (optional)

- "Software"

  — Barbed broaches—used to remove pulp
  — Gates Glidden drills
  — Endodontic files—diameter sizes 10–80, length sizes 21, 25, and 55 mm
  — Paper points—for drying canal, same sizes and diameters as files
  — Gutta-percha—inert filling material for root canal

— Zinc oxide–eugenol liquid paste sealer for root apex
— Pluggers and spreaders
— Glass ionomer cement
— Composite or amalgam for restoration

Procedure for Root Canal Therapy

Step one—Accessing the canal(s): Often, the access hole will be premade from the fracture. Other times, you will have to make another hole to line up with the pulp chamber to avoid bending the endodontic files (Fig. 7.46). Cat and small dog teeth are usually entered from the fracture site.

Step two—Preparing the canal(s) (preparation):

1. Gates Glidden drills are used to widen the canal (Fig. 7.47).
2. A barbed broach is used to hook the pulp for removal of part or whole (Fig. 7.48).

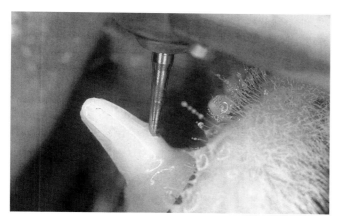

Fig. 7.46. Access entrance is made midcrown.

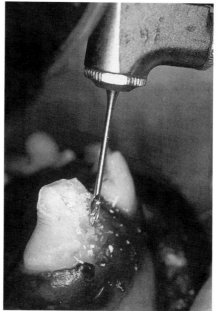

Fig. 7.47. Widening the root canal with the Gates Glidden drill.

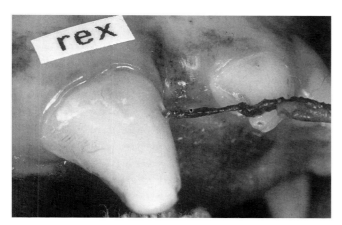

Fig. 7.48. Necrotic pulp extracted with help of a barbed broach.

3. Files are used to shape and clean the canal (Fig. 7.49). With the introduction of a larger file, the canal is irrigated with sodium hypochlorite. This process is called **debridement**.

4. A radiograph is taken with file in place to verify the file is at the root apex of the tooth (Fig. 7.50).

5. The working length (length of file from access to apex) is determined by radiography. A rubber stop is placed on the file to make sure the proper length is filed. The stop prevents the file from harming periapical tissues.

6. When the veterinarian is satisfied with canal preparation, the canal is irrigated with sterile saline and dried by placing sterile paper points into the opening of the tooth. The tooth is now ready to be filled and sealed.

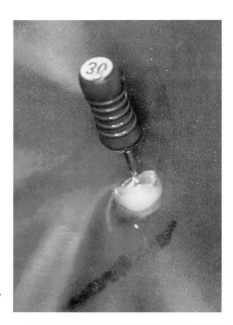

Fig. 7.49. File inside root canal.

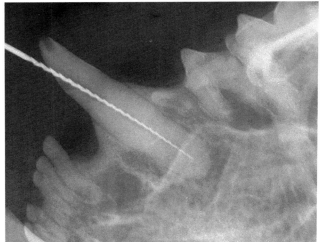

Fig. 7.50. Radiograph taken to confirm file is at apex.

Step three—Filling and sealing the root canal(s) (obturation):

1. A gutta-percha trial point (master cone) is placed into the pulp chamber to the apex and radiographed to confirm the gutta-percha reaches the apex. The cone is removed.

2. Zinc oxide–eugenol cement is prepared on a sterile glass slab.

3. The cement is either loaded on a Lentulo spiral filler, applied with an endodontic file, or placed on the apex of additional gutta-percha points to seal the root apex (Fig. 7.51).

4. The master cone and additional gutta-percha points are placed in the canal.

5. Pluggers and spreaders, beginning with the widest and progressing to smaller sizes, are used to compact the gutta-percha points in the canal until full.

Step four—Restoring the tooth (restoration):

1. With an inverted cone or pear bur, 2–3 mm of the filled gutta-percha is removed from the coronal portion of the canal.

2. Calcium hydroxide or glass ionomer cement is used as an intermediate restorative on top of the gutta-percha and below the composite restorative.

3. The composite restorative is placed and cured.

4. The restorative is polished.

5. If a metallic or porcelain crown is planned, the tooth is prepared for impression.

Figures 7.52 and 7.53 are radiographs taken before and after root canal therapy.

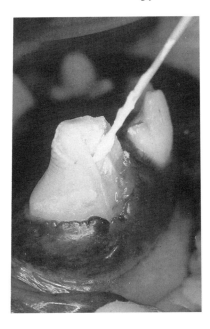

Fig. 7.51. Zinc oxide-eugenol is placed on tip of a gutta-percha point before being placed into canal.

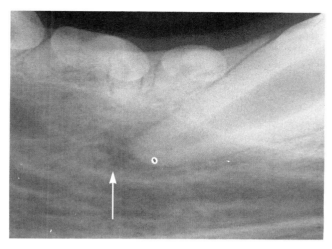

Fig. 7.52. *Preoperative radiograph revealing a periapical lucency* (arrow) *in a one-and-one-half-year-old German shepherd.*

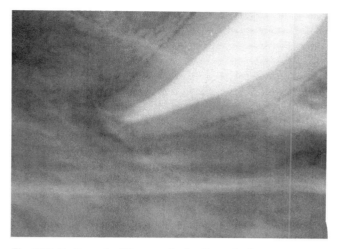

Fig. 7.53. *Radiograph of German shepherd's tooth after root canal therapy.*

Endodontic Therapy Depending on the Age of the Patient

The root apex closes between 12 and 18 months. Conventional root canal therapy must not be done on those animals with an open apex because sealing the root canal cannot be ensured. Based on the health of the pulp, apexogenesis or apexification can be performed to care for a young animal's fractured tooth.

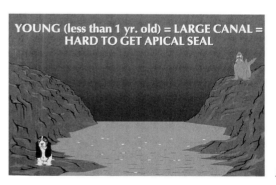

Fig. 7.54.

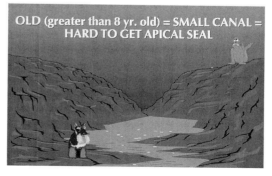

Fig. 7.55.

Animals 8 years old and older will have a very thin canal, requiring additional time to remove and fill the pulp chamber.

APEXOGENESIS

If the fracture is recent (less than two weeks old) *and* the patient is less than one and a half years old, apexogenesis (vital pulpotomy) can be performed (Figs. 7.56–7.59). The goal of apexogenesis in the acutely traumatized tooth of a young animal is to permit closure of the root apex, allowing for future conventional endodontics, while stimulating secondary dentin at the fracture site to protect the pulp. Apexogenesis of a fractured tooth in an eight-month-old puppy is shown in Figures 7.57 and 7.58.

- One to 4 mm of pulp tissue are removed with a high-speed drill.

- A direct pulp cap with calcium hydroxide is applied as a dressing on top of the vital pulp. Calcium hydroxide stimulates dentinogenesis, the forming of a new seal (called a dentinal bridge) over the fracture site. Hopefully, the tooth will remain vital and continue to grow, eventually leading to a sealed apex.

- The tooth is restored with acrylic bonding.

- Radiographs are taken at three-month intervals. If there is any evidence of periapical pathology after the apex closes, conventional or surgical endodontics is performed.

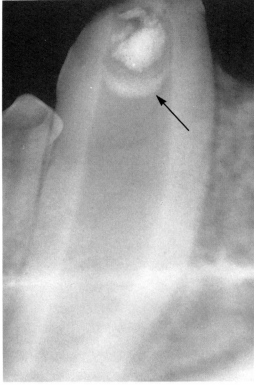

Fig. 7.56. *Radiograph of apexo-genesis with creation of dentinal bridge* (arrow).

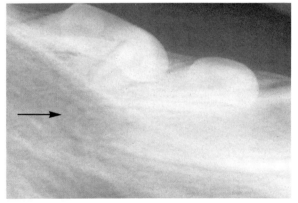

Fig. 7.57. *Radiograph of preoperative open root apex in fractured tooth of eight-month-old puppy* (arrow).

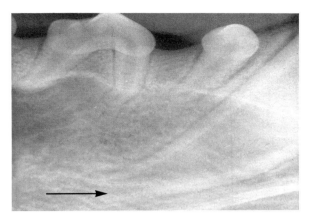

Fig. 7.58. *Radiograph of successful apexogenesis in creating a closed root apex* (arrow).

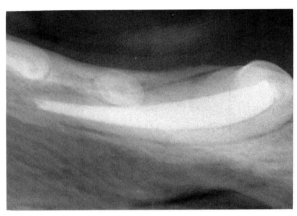

Fig. 7.59. *Radiograph of conventional root canal to seal apex once apex closed.*

APEXIFICATION

Apexification is performed on partially developed permanent teeth in which pulpal inflammation and necrosis have occurred to the point where preservation of the pulp is no longer possible. Calcium hydroxide is used to stimulate the periapical tissues to create a bony closure of the root apex.

Apexification is accomplished by performing conventional endodontics with the exception that calcium hydroxide paste is used to fill the canal. Follow-up radiographs are taken every two months to evaluate apical closure. The calcium hydroxide needs to be replaced every two to three months. Once the apex is closed, the calcium hydroxide is removed, and the canal filled with gutta-percha and zinc oxide–eugenol.

Endodontic Therapy Requiring Surgery (Apicoectomy)

An **apicoectomy** with retrograde filling is performed when

- Teeth have periapical infections that do not respond to conventional endodontic therapy.
- There are unretrievable file tip fractures at the beginning of a conventional endodontic procedure.
- A horizontal distal root fracture is present with periapical pathology.
- The veterinarian is unable to perfect an apical seal due to obstruction.

MATERIALS FOR SURGICAL ENDODONTICS

- A high- and low-speed delivery system
- Burs (crosscut fissure, round, and inverted)
- Periosteal elevator
- Suture kit
- Centrix syringe
- Retrograde carrier
- Gutta-percha, intermediate restorative material (IRM), restorative

SURGICAL ENDODONTIC PROCEDURE

- Conventional endodontics is performed.

- A semilunar incision is made over the affected root apex. The periosteum is elevated around the apex.

- Bone overlying the apex is drilled, exposing 5 mm circumferentially.

- The apex is amputated using a crosscut fissure bur. Gutta-percha condensed from conventional endodontics should be observed.

- An inverted cone bur is used to undercut the access site 2–3 mm. Intermediate restorative material (IRM), Super EBA (Bisco), or zinc-free amalgam is applied to seal the apex.

- The flap is closed.

ENDODONTIC-PERIODONTIC LESIONS

Some small animals suffer from both endodontic and periodontic lesions in the same tooth (Fig. 7.60). Communication from the pulp to periodontal support can come from the tooth's root apex or lateral canals.

To be classified as an endodontic-periodontic lesion, there must be at least one root with a necrotic pulp and destruction of the periodontal attachment extending from either the gingival sulcus or lateral canal to the apex.

Therapy options depend on the degree of periodontal involvement. In cases of minor involvement, conventional or surgical endodontics and antibiotics will be curative. Where attachment loss is marked, extraction of the tooth or hemisection of the affected root plus endodontics on the remaining root(s) is the treatment of choice (Fig. 7.61).

CROWN THERAPY

Crowns are placed on top of fractured teeth to provide additional fracture and wear protection. Materials chosen for crown restoration depend on how the crown was fractured and the oral habits of the dog or cat. An acrylic composite is easy to apply as a restoration and approximates the appearance of the tooth (Fig. 7.62).

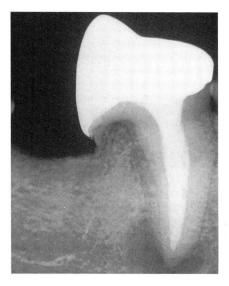

Fig. 7.61. Radiograph of hemisected endodontically treated tooth three months postoperative. Note the filled in bone in the area occupied by the distal root.

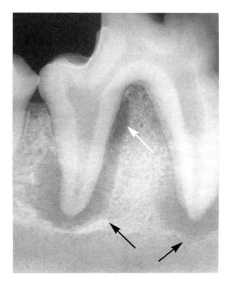

Fig. 7.60. Radiograph of endodontic-periodontic lesion. White arrow points to periodontic lesion; black arrows point to endodontic lesions.

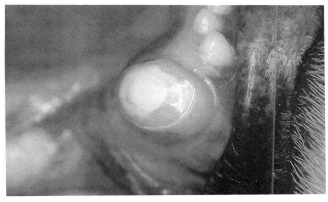

Fig. 7.62. Acrylic restoration of fracture site.

Unfortunately, due to marginal leakage and fracture, acrylic does not hold up well to long-term occlusal trauma. A better choice for restoration is metallic crowns fabricated from nickel and chromium (Fig. 7.63). Porcelain is another restorative choice, but it chips easily and should not be used in animals that are prone to chew on hard objects (Figs. 7.64 and 7.65).

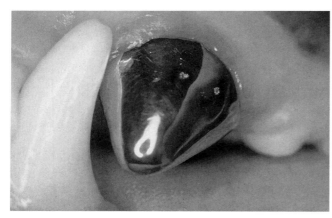

Fig. 7.63. Metallic crown restoration.

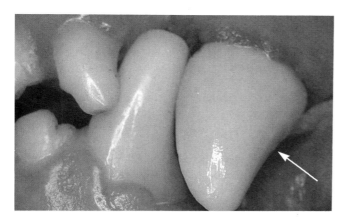

Fig. 7.64. Porcelain crown restoration (arrow).

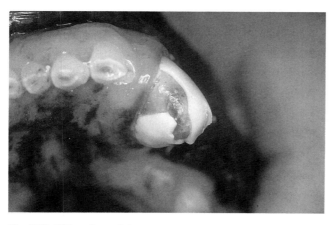

Fig. 7.65. Chipped porcelain crown.

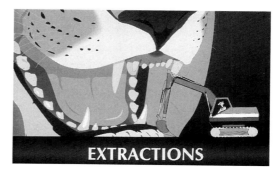

Fig. 7.66.

EXTRACTION
Extraction is the most common oral surgical procedure performed.

Indications for Extraction

- Periodontal disease where greater than 50 percent of the bone is lost and the owner does not agree (1) to surgery to try to save the tooth and/or (2) to perform postoperative oral hygiene

- Fractured tooth with pulpal exposure, where the owner will not consent to endodontic therapy

- Abscess formation from endodontic or periodontal disease, where the owner will not consent to therapy

- Malpositioned teeth caused by retained primary teeth or overcrowding resulting in food impaction, periodontal disease, trauma to adjacent teeth and tissues, or trauma to teeth and tissues in the opposing arch

- Jaw fractures through the alveolus

Extraction Tips
To perform an extraction, knowledge of dental anatomy is a must. Especially important is knowing the number of roots and root lengths for each tooth.
Some anatomical guides:

- The shortest rooted **incisors** are the centrals; the longest rooted are the laterals. Roots curve laterally with the maxillary apices a few millimeters from the nasal cavity.

- Maxillary **canines** lie within 2 mm of the nasal cavity. Care should be taken not to apply medial or palatal force. Flap exposure and removal of the overlying alveolar bone facilitate extraction.

- The **first premolar** has only one root.

- The **second and third maxillary premolars** have two roots and should be hemisected to convert to two single-rooted teeth for extraction. The distal root apex of the third premolar lies close to the infraorbital foramen.

- The **fourth maxillary premolar** has three roots (two large buccal and one smaller palatal). Sectioning into three single roots facilitates extraction.

- The **first and second maxillary molars** have three roots in a tripod arrangement.

- **Mandibular canines, premolars,** and **molars** are encased in thick bone. This bony support presents considerable resistance to tooth extraction. Use of heavy force can result in a tooth or mandibular fracture.

- **All mandibular premolars and molars distal to the first premolar** have two roots.

Figure 7.67 depicts maxillary premolar and first molar teeth sectioned into one-rooted segments.

Preoperative radiographs are taken for two reasons:

- To identify abnormal root or periapical structures
- For record-keeping reasons to document the reason for extraction

Extraction Procedure

- The coronal portion of the periodontal ligament is severed with a scalpel blade.

- **Luxators** are elevators used to help remove teeth (Fig. 7.68). The blade end is placed between the root and alveolar bone or between sectioned crowns.

- Rocking the luxator blade back and forth will not aid in extraction. Holding the luxator with moderate axial torque *for 30–60 seconds* in a single direction will eventually fatigue the periodontal ligament, gently lifting the tooth from the alveolar socket.

- Dental forceps are aligned with the long axis of the tooth to lift it from the oral cavity. The choice of forceps used is important. Most human forceps do not grasp dogs' or cats' teeth adequately. Use of improperly sized forceps can lead to fracture of the tooth or alveolus. The forceps' beaks must be in full contact with the tooth. Rongeurs can be used successfully.

Forceps must not be used as an extracting instrument. Brute torquing force will either fracture the tooth, alveolar socket, or jaw. If the tooth is not mobile enough for gentle lifting, then more time is necessary for applying the luxator to fatigue the periodontal ligament.

- If the tooth still does not budge, a flap procedure is performed to expose the facial alveolar plate. A high-speed drill with a round bur is used to remove the lateral plate, making the extraction easier.

Surgical extraction via flap exposure is the preferred method for removing canines, maxillary fourth premolars, mandibular molars, retained roots, and other multirooted teeth for which nonsurgical exposure does not result in an easy extraction.

Vertical incisions are made along the interdental spaces on either side of the tooth to be extracted. The attached gingiva is reflected with the help of a periosteal elevator.

A high-speed bur is used to remove part of the lateral alveolus to facilitate extraction. The luxator is used in the space between the alveolus and tooth to dislodge the tooth. Following extraction, the alveolar ridge is smoothed out (alveolarplasty) with a round bur prior to suturing.

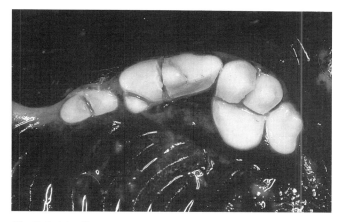

Fig. 7.67. Maxillary premolar and first molar teeth sectioned into one-rooted segments.

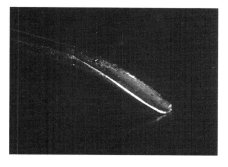

Fig. 7.68. Luxator tip.

Figures 7.69–7.72 depict extraction of a mandibular first molar affected by grade four periodontal disease. Regardless of the method used for extraction, inspect the tooth to ensure the entire root has been removed. The root apex, when fully extracted, will appear as a smooth, rounded surface. If you see a ragged apex, part of the root remains and must be removed from the alveolus. Often flap exposure and removal of the lateral alveolar plate over the root tip will be necessary to find and remove the root fragment.

Some practitioners feel they need to fill the void left from the extracted tooth. Tetracycline powder, gelatin sponge, cancellous harvested bone, as well as Bioglass have been used in the past. Unless the defect appears to limit the patient's ability to eat comfortably, the void created does not need to be filled with an implant. In time, the defect will fill with cancellous bone.

HEMISECTION TO SAVE PART OF A TOOTH

The second through fourth premolars and all molars are multirooted teeth. Often, some roots are affected with disease and cannot be saved, but efforts can be made to save remaining roots and provide a functional tooth.

Indications for hemisection include

- Endodontic reasons (separated instruments, root perforations from resorption, obstructed canals, marked internal resorption)
- Periodontal reasons (F3 furcation involvement or bone loss greater than 50 percent on some of the tooth's roots but not all)

Sectioning is performed with a 701L crosscut fissure bur. A gingival flap may be necessary for hemisection to gain access to the root. If the root is affected with marked bone loss, the flap is usually not necessary. The hemisection cut should not divide the tooth directly in half but should be 1–3 mm away from the root to be sacrificed.

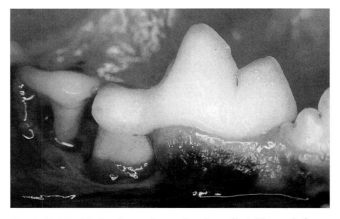

Fig. 7.69. Mandibular first and second molars affected by grade four periodontal disease.

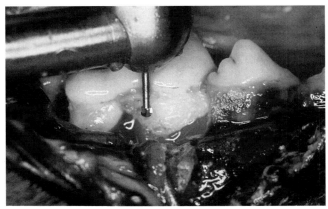

Fig. 7.70. First molar's roots exposed by flap surgery. A high-speed drill is used to section tooth.

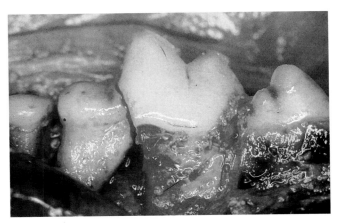

Fig. 7.71. Hemisection to convert the two-rooted first molar into two single-rooted sections.

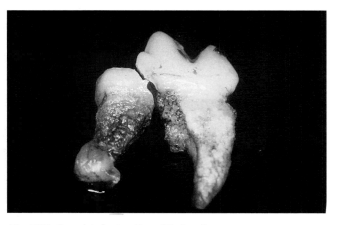

Fig. 7.72. Completed extraction of first molar.

✑Endodontic Care at a Glance

Problem	Appearance	Treatment
Enamel fracture	Nick or gouge on enamel surface	Radiographs to confirm no periapical lesion, defect smoothed out with white stone
Enamel and dentin fracture	Yellow dentin exposed	Radiographs as above; if pulp noted on visual examination, indirect pulp dentin capping performed; if not noted, radiographs every six months to check for endodontic lesions. Antibiotics and pain medication pre-/postoperatively
Enamel and dentin fracture, pulp exposed	Pulp visible as either red dot (recent fracture) or black penetrating hole into pulp chamber (chronic fracture)	Apexogenesis (vital pulpotomy) if pet is under 18 months and tooth is vital; apexification if tooth is infected and apex is open. Conventional endodontics if pet is over 18 months. Surgical endodontics if apex is not sealable conventionally. Antibiotics and pain medication pre-/postoperatively
Recent fracture exposing pulp (within 48 hours)	Bleeding or red dot noted in center of tooth	Vital pulpotomy or conventional endodontics
Endodontic-periodontic lesions	Abscess noted above and below the mucogingival line or fractured tooth that is also mobile	If the tooth can be saved, first treat for endodontic disease, wait for healing, then address the periodontal problems.
Pulpitis	Discolored tooth (off-white, pink, purple, brown, gray)	Radiograph and conventional or surgical endodontics if the patient is older than 18 months
Avulsed tooth	Tooth out of socket due to trauma	Owner instructed to put tooth in milk and refer dog to veterinarian with expertise in stabilization and root canal therapy

FELINE DENTAL PATHOLOGY AND CARE

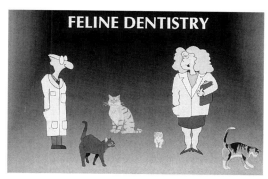

Fig. 7.73.

Feline dental pathology is perhaps the most overlooked and undertreated area in small animal medicine. Greater than 65 percent of feline patients over five years old have oral lesions that require immediate care to relieve pain.

Feline Odontoclastic Resorptive Lesions

One of the most perplexing cat oral problems is called the feline odontoclastic resorptive lesion (FORL). FORLs are tooth defects that have also been called

- Cavities
- Neck lesions

- External or internal root resorptions
- External odontoclastic resorptions
- Cervical line erosions

The location of a FORL is usually at the labial or buccal surface near the cemento-enamel junction (CEJ) where the free gingiva meets the tooth surface. The teeth most commonly affected are the mandibular third premolar and first molars and maxillary third and fourth premolars; however, FORLs can be found on any tooth (Fig. 7.74).

The etiology is unknown; however, theories supporting an autoimmune response mediating cellular and humoral factors, calicivirus, and metabolic imbalances relating to calcium regulation have been proposed.

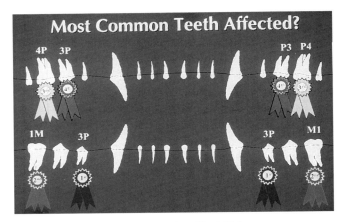

Fig. 7.74. Teeth most commonly affected by FORLs.

Patients affected with FORLs may show hypersalivation, oral bleeding, or difficulty eating food. *A majority of affected cats do not show clinical signs.* It is usually up to the clinician or technician to diagnose the lesions on oral examination.

Clinically, resorptions are areas where tooth substance is missing. Diagnostic aids include a periodontal probe or cotton-tipped applicator applied to the suspected FORL. The lesion often erodes into sensitive dentin, causing the cat to show pain with jaw spasms when the FORL is touched.

Intraoral radiology is helpful in making a definitive diagnosis and for treatment planning. The radiographic appearance of FORLs varies from minute radiolucent defects of the tooth at the cemento-enamel junction to internal resorption and ankylosis of the root apex to the supporting bone.

The FORL can present in many stages:

- In the **class one FORL,** an enamel defect is noted. The lesion is minimally sensitive because it has not entered dentin. Therapy for this defect involves thorough cleaning and polishing. Gingivectomy and odontoplasty have also been used. Pulse therapy antibiotics aid in controlling plaque accumulation in all stages of FORLs and may be helpful. In addition, periodic application of fluoride toothpaste is advocated for decreasing pain and plaque.

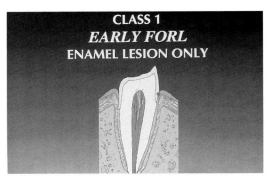

Fig. 7.75.

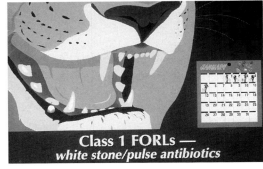

Fig. 7.76.

- **Class two FORLs** penetrate the enamel and dentin (Fig. 7.78). Intraoral radiography is essential to determine if the lesions have entered the pulp chamber. Class two FORLs are painful and must be treated by extraction or glass ionomer restoration.

The class two FORL may be treated with a self- or light-cured glass ionomer restorative, which releases fluoride ions to desensitize the exposed dentin, strengthens the enamel, and chemically binds to the tooth surface. (A class two FORL treated with a glass ionomer restoration is shown in Figs. 7.79 and 7.80.) The long-term (greater than two years) effectiveness of restoration of class two lesions is poor (<10%). Glass ionomer application to the FORL does not automatically stop progression of disease.

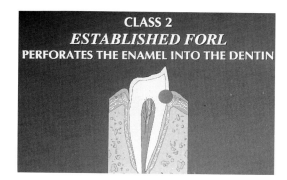

Fig. 7.77.

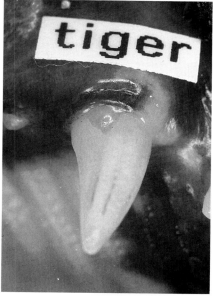

Fig. 7.79. Class two FORL.

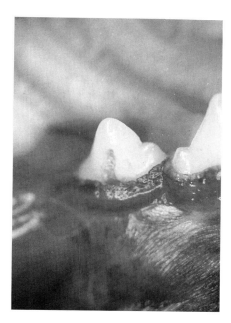

Fig. 7.78. *Class two FORL.*

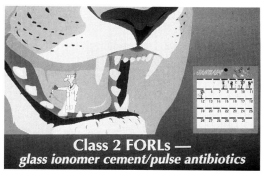

Fig. 7.80. *Class two FORL treated with glass ionomer restoration.*

The class two FORL treatment procedure with self-cured glass ionomer follows:

1. The area to be treated is first cleaned with a curette or scaler. Flour pumice and water is used as a polish (not prophy paste).

2. The gingiva is isolated by packing with gingival retraction cord.

3. The area is irrigated and dried (not bone dry).

4. Class two glass ionomers are used for FORL restorations. Once mixed, the glass ionomer cement is placed on top of the lesion. When set, a varnish or nonfilled light-cured resin is placed over the restoration.

5. The restoration is then finished and shaped using a finishing bur. A second coat of varnish or

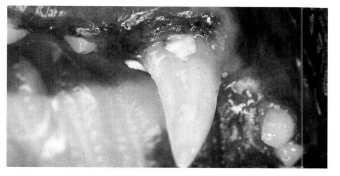

Fig. 7.81.

resin is placed over the restoration to maintain proper moisture levels while curing.

- **Class three FORLs** enter the endodontic system (Fig. 7.83). These lesions require either extraction or endodontics to seal the canal from oral bacteria.

Restoration with glass ionomer restoratives is not an option. Intraoral radiology is a must to evaluate the root before considering therapy.

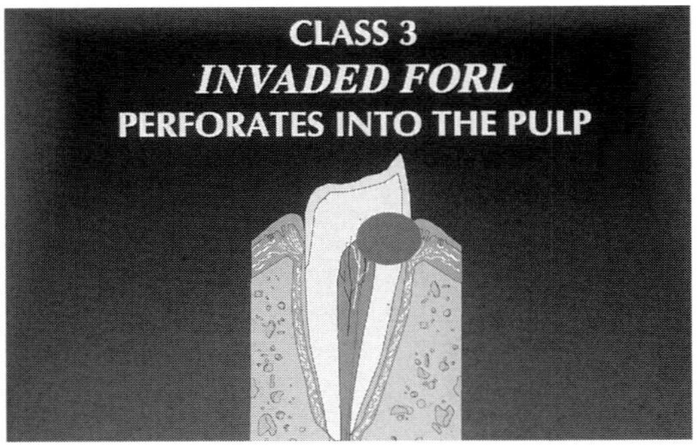

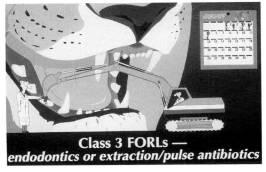

Fig. 7.82.

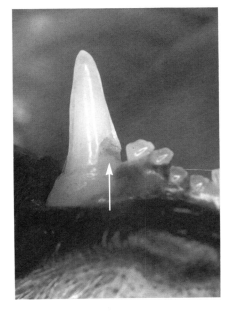

Fig. 7.83. Class three FORL (arrow).

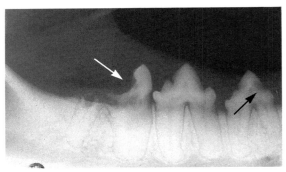

Fig. 7.84.

• In the **class four** FORL, the crown has been eroded or fractured, leaving part of the crown exposed (Figs. 7.86 and 7.87). Gingiva grows over the root

fragments, leaving a sensitive and often bleeding lesion upon probing. Treatment of choice is flap surgery to extract the root fragments.

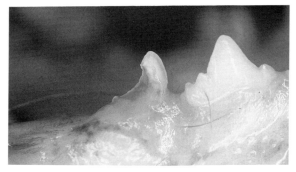

Fig. 7.85.

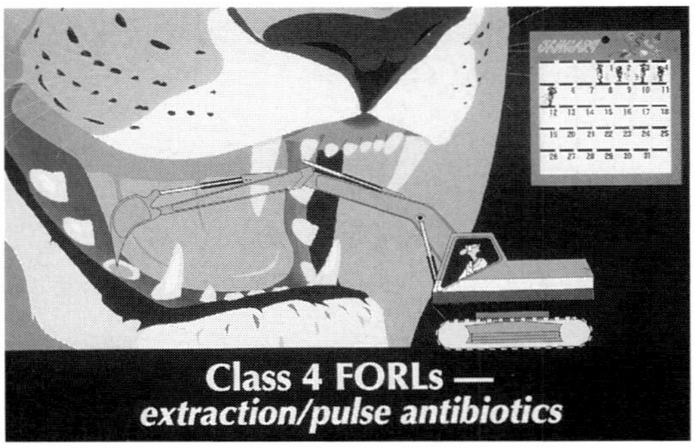

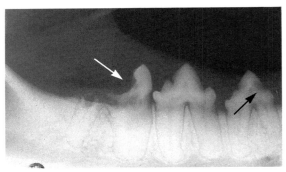

Fig. 7.88.

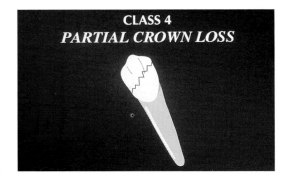

Fig. 7.86. Class four FORL.

Fig. 7.87. Radiograph of FORLs. Class three on third premolar (black arrow) and class four on first molar (white arrow).

• In the **class five FORL**, the crown is gone, but radiographs indicate roots remain (Fig. 7.90). The decision whether or not to perform flap surgery to find and extract the retained roots is based on pain. If the cat feels discomfort when the lesion is probed, then the roots are extracted.

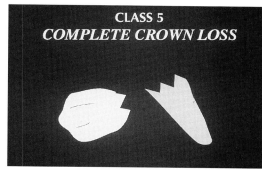

Fig. 7.89.

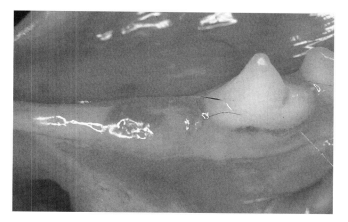

Fig. 7.90. Class five FORL.

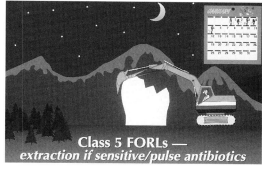

Fig. 7.91.

Lymphocytic Plasmacytic Gingivitis Stomatitis

Cats can also be affected by stomatitis (generalized inflammation of the mouth), more specifically referred to as LPGS (lymphocytic plasmacytic gingivitis stomatitis). The etiology of this disease has not been determined. An immune-related cause is suspected due to the large number of plasma cells on histopathology.

Gingival signs of LPGS in affected cats include

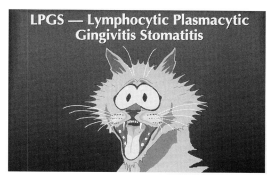

Fig. 7.92.

• Dysphagia
• Weight loss
• Ptyalism

Signs of LPGS found in an oral examination include

• Faucitis, a "cobblestonelike" hyperplasia and hyperemia on the glossopalatine and palatopharyngeal arches, soft palate, and oropharynx—present in one-third of the LPGS-affected patients (Fig. 7.93)

• Marked gingivitis and periodontitis around the premolars and molars

• Moderate to severe periodontal disease with bone loss

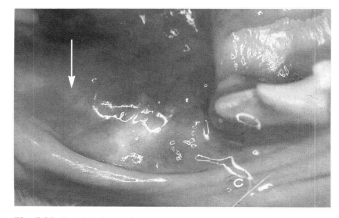

Fig. 7.93. Faucitis (arrow).

- All stages of feline odontoclastic resorptive lesions can also be apparent clinically and radiographically.

Traditional therapy options for LPGS include

- Thorough cleaning and polishing
- Gingivectomy
- Corticosteroids
- Gold salts
- Metronidazole
- Megestrol acetate
- Laser

Unfortunately, most nonextraction therapeutic approaches will not lead to long-term success. If the syndrome is due to a hyperimmune response to the tooth, then most therapies short of extraction will fail.

An effective approach to diagnosis and care for LPGS is

- First, rule in or out other internal medical problems. Feline leukemia and feline immunodeficiency virus should be checked for, and a chemical profile and urinalysis for metabolic abnormalities should be performed. Expect high gamma globulin results due to the chronicity of LPGS.

- Intraoral radiographs are taken of all the teeth and gingival areas of missing teeth. With the radiographic findings, each tooth can then be examined and treated individually.

- If a tooth is affected by moderate to severe periodontitis typified by greater than 50 percent bone loss, it should be extracted. In addition, all root fragments need to be removed. Radiographs are repeated after extraction to ensure complete tooth removal.

- In severe cases all teeth distal to the canines are extracted (Figs. 7.94 and 7.95).

- Immediately following surgery, prednisone (1 mm/lb) is given daily and tapered over a 10-day period.

- Starting two weeks after surgery, the client is advised and shown how to daily brush the cat's remaining teeth. Daily toothbrushing should be followed by irrigation with 0.2 percent chlorhexidine.

- If the above treatment does not work within two months, then all remaining teeth are removed.

- About 20 percent of cases will still have lesions and will partially respond to lifelong medical therapy.

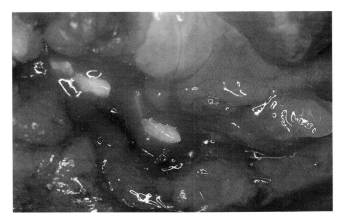

Fig. 7.94. LPGS. Note marked inflammation.

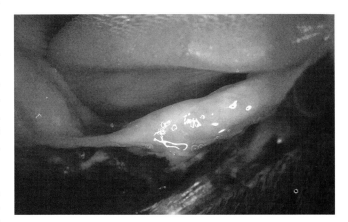

Fig. 7.95. Resolution of LPGS inflammation after extraction of all teeth distal to canines.

Cancer

Not all feline oral swellings are malignant. Cats are frequently affected by treatable oral foreign body granulomatous reactions, osteomyelitis (deep bone infections) arising from dental or traumatic disease, eosinophilic granulomas, fungal infections, and nasopharyngeal polyps. Biopsies are essential because the clinical appearance of malignancy can be deceiving.

Squamous cell carcinoma (SCC) is the most prevalent type of oral cancer. SCC can arise from the oral epithelium and is characterized by local extension and invasion. Morbidity and mortality come from local disease rather than distant metastasis. Less common feline oral malignancies include

- Melanoma
- Fibrosarcoma
- Lymphosarcoma
- Osteosarcoma
- Undifferentiated carcinomas

☞ Feline Dental Care at a Glance

Problem	Appearance	Treatment
Class one FORL	Minimal enamel penetration, minimal gingival inflammation	Radiographs to closer examine crown and root for additional resorptions, gingivectomy over lesion, odontoplasty to smooth out lesion, owner instructed to brush with fluoride toothpaste. Pulse therapy antibiotics
Class two FORL	Lesion enters dentin but not pulp	Radiography as above. If lesion has not entered pulp, glass ionomer cement can be applied to FORL. Pulse therapy antibiotics
Class three FORL	Lesion enters pulp	If canine tooth, maxillary fourth premolar, or mandibular first molar, then consider endodontics when radiographs confirm an apical seal can be perfected. If not, then extraction via flap surgery. Pulse therapy antibiotics
Class four FORL	Lesion has destroyed part of crown	Extraction via flap surgery. Pulse therapy antibiotics
Class five FORL	Lesion has destroyed all of the crown. A swelling is noted on the gingiva.	If the patient experiences pain via the applicator test, then extract the retained root(s). If not and the radiographs do not reveal periapical lesions, reradiograph three to six months later.
Feline lymphocytic plasmacytic gingivitis stomatitis (LPGS) syndrome	Circumferential inflammation around all teeth, faucitis	Preoperative testing for feline leukemia (FELV) and feline immunodeficiency virus (FIV), radiology and extraction of all teeth with greater than 50 percent bone loss, postoperative antibiotics, pain medication and tapering dosages of corticosteroids. If poor response, extract teeth distal to canines or extract all teeth.

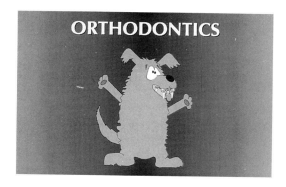

Fig. 7.96.

ORAL CONDITIONS REQUIRING ORTHODONTIC CARE

Braces for animals? Sure! Just as you would treat a painful skin condition or sore joint, you must also relieve pain in a pet's mouth brought on by orthodontic abnormalities. Poorly aligned teeth can lead to periodontal disease, tooth loss, and penetrating gingival injury.

In most breeds, teeth are arranged in the arch "shoulder to shoulder." A self-cleaning mechanism pushes food away from the teeth and gums. If teeth are not aligned normally, food is retained between the teeth, often causing inflammation and infection. Deviated teeth can also be painful for the pet when penetration of gum tissue occurs.

The normal alignment of the maxilla and mandible of dogs and cats with medium to long muzzles is called a **scissors bite** (Fig. 7.97). In the scissors bite

- Maxillary incisors are just in front of the mandibular incisors when the mouth is closed.

- The mandibular canine crown lies equally between the maxillary lateral incisor and maxillary canine and touches neither.

- Premolar crown tips point to a space between the crowns of the opposing premolars.

In dogs that have a short and wide muzzle, a **reverse scissors**, or underbite, is considered normal. Mandibular incisors are in front of the maxillary incisors. Mandibular canines and premolars are shifted forward.

Is the Orthodontic Problem Genetic or Not?

Not all orthodontic abnormalities are caused by genetic defects. Occlusion is controlled by

- Genetics
- Traumatic birthing
- Nutrition
- Environment
- Mechanical forces generated by an interlock of the maxillary and mandibular teeth

Retained deciduous teeth cause numerous orthodontic problems. Tug-of-war games with towels or ropes can also move teeth into abnormal positions and must be avoided.

To define if the problem is genetic in origin, the interdigitation of the premolars is studied. In the normal medium or long muzzled dog or cat, premolars meet in a saw-toothed fashion, where the tips of the mandibular premolars point to the spaces between their maxillary counterparts—that is, the tip of the mandibular third premolar should be positioned equally between the crowns of the maxillary third and fourth premolars

(Fig 7.98). If the tip of one premolar points at the tip of another, the malocclusion probably has a genetic etiology (Fig. 7.99).

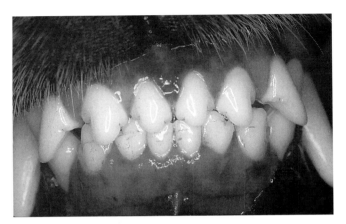

Fig. 7.97. Scissors bite (normal occlusion).

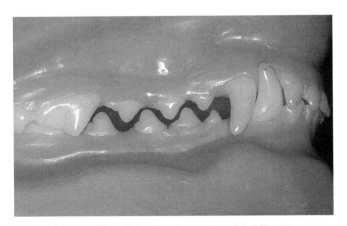

Fig. 7.98. Normal interdigitation of premolars. (Model by Henry Schein, Inc.).

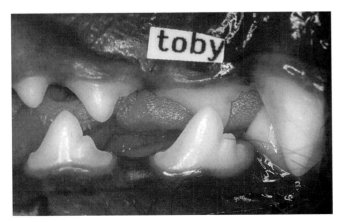

Fig. 7.99. Genetic malocclusion—poor premolar interdigitation.

Retained Deciduous Teeth

As a general rule, any time there is an abnormality caused by deciduous teeth (Fig. 7.100), those teeth causing the problem are extracted under general anesthesia. For example, Figures 7.101–7.103 depict the extraction of mandibular deciduous canines that are penetrating the maxilla. Progress reexams are a must to make sure that the adult canines do not also cause problems necessitating orthodontic care.

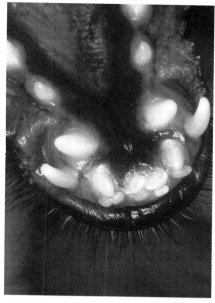

Fig. 7.100. Retained deciduous teeth.

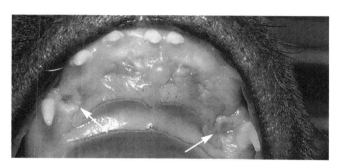

Fig. 7.101. Mandibular deciduous canine penetrating into maxilla.

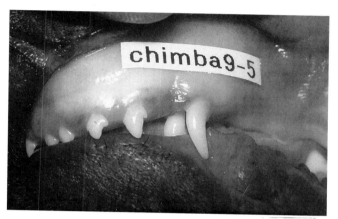

Fig. 7.102. Maxilla showing penetration areas palatal to canines (arrows).

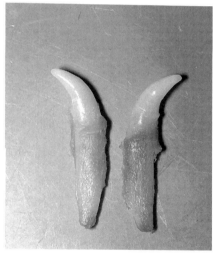

Fig. 7.103. Extracted mandibular deciduous canines.

Retained primary teeth mainly occur in smaller breeds, especially Maltese, Yorkshire terriers, poodles, and miniature schnauzers. Normally, the deciduous tooth's root is resorbed, making room for the adult tooth. When this fails, the adult tooth deviates from its normal position (Fig. 7.104). The double set of teeth overcrowds the dental arch, and food can become trapped between teeth, causing gingivitis. The double set of roots may also prevent normal development of the socket and periodontal support around the adult tooth, resulting in early tooth loss. A retained deciduous tooth must be extracted as soon as the adult tooth

erupts in the same socket. If extraction is performed early, the abnormally positioned adult tooth usually moves to its normal location.

A common procedure performed by some breeders is to "trim" the deciduous teeth in the hope that they will be shed early, thus preventing orthodontic problems. By cutting the tooth in half, the nerve and blood supply is exposed to the oral environment, eventually causing an infection and tooth loss. Trimming is not a recommended procedure because it results in pain for the animal and the inflammation caused can affect the adjoining adult teeth.

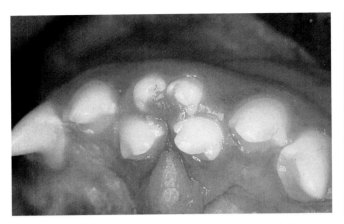

Fig. 7.104. Retained maxillary incisor deciduous teeth displacing central incisors distally.

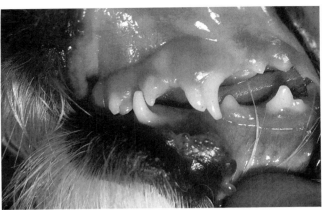

Fig. 7.105. Dental interlock. Note mandibular canine locking maxillary incisors, preventing forward growth. Treatment consists of extracting mandibular deciduous canines.

Dental Interlock

The maxilla and mandible do not grow at equal rates. When deciduous teeth erupt during an accelerated growth phase of one jaw, an interlocking of both sets of deciduous teeth can maintain an abnormal bite relationship (Fig. 7.105). Even genetically normal dogs can occasionally develop abnormal bites due to the interlock of deciduous teeth.

In a breed that normally has a scissors bite, the young puppy or kitten with an underbite may respond to treatment if the animal's permanent teeth have not yet erupted. On the shorter jaw, primary teeth impeding forward growth are removed by the time the patient is 12 weeks old. This procedure, called **interceptive orthodontics**, allows correction of about 10 percent of interlocked malocclusions by the time permanent teeth erupt. The extraction does nothing to stimulate jaw growth; it removes the mechanical barrier to genetic control of the growth process.

Teeth that are crowded, rotated, or tilted at abnormal angles can result in

- Early onset and increased severity of oral infection

- Damage to the soft tissues of the mouth due to sharp teeth penetrating unprotected gingiva. Mandibular canines can erode the hard palate, causing food to enter the nasal cavity.

- Excessive wear when abnormally aligned teeth grind against each other. This abrasion frequently wears through enamel, causing a weakened tooth to fracture and expose the root canal system.

- Pain in the joints of the jaw as well as in the gums, lips, cheeks, and teeth

Missing or Extra Teeth

Dogs and cats may be born without the proper number of teeth. Extra (**supernumerary**) teeth can cause periodontal disease from overcrowding and should be extracted. The American Kennel Club sets standards concerning the minimum number of teeth for many breeds of dog that are shown.

Dental radiographs can be taken as early as 10 weeks of age to evaluate if the correct number teeth are present. Dental radiographs are recommended as a part of the prepurchase examination of certain breeds to be used for show.

Missing teeth (**hypodontia**) are usually recognized in the incisor or premolar areas, but any tooth in the mouth may be missing. Missing teeth are considered genetic faults. Collies and Doberman pinschers are most commonly affected. Sometimes, the missing tooth is present below the gum line. A radiograph is taken to determine if there is a nonerupted (**impacted**) tooth. Removal of gingiva covering the tooth may permit it to erupt, as shown in Figures 7.106–7.109.

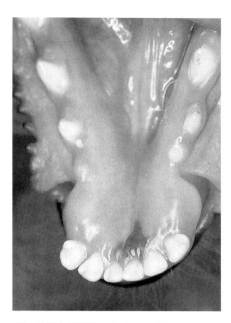

Fig. 7.106. Visibly missing canines.

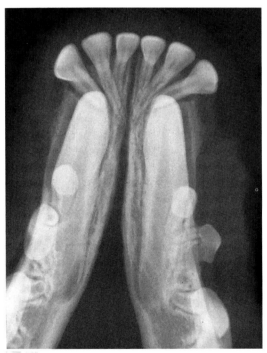

Fig. 7.107. Radiograph showing unerupted canines.

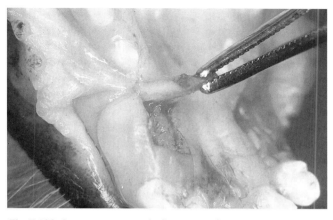

Fig. 7.108. Surgery to remove gingiva over canines.

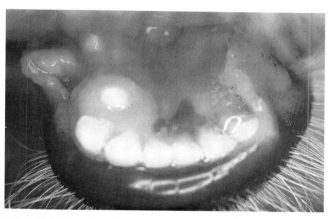

Fig. 7.109. Erupted canine.

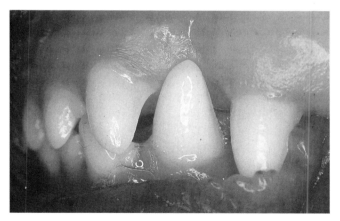

Fig. 7.110. Normal occlusion. Note equal space between the mandibular canine and maxillary canine and lateral incisor.

Malocclusion

Malocclusion refers to abnormal tooth alignment. This can occur from a skeletal problem where one jaw is longer or shorter than it should be or from a dental problem where teeth are not aligned normally even though the jaw lengths are normal.

Overbite is a term used by breeders and veterinarians to describe an extension of the maxillary teeth in front of the mandibular dentition (Fig. 7.111). (In the pure sense, an overbite is a vertical malocclusion. For the purpose of this book, we will use the generally accepted orthodontic terms rather than the purely scientific ones.) With an overbite, the maxillary premolars are displaced at least 25 percent forward compared with the mandibular premolars. There may be a gap between the maxillary and mandibular incisors when the mouth is closed. An overbite has also been (somewhat incorrectly) referred to as

- Overshot
- Parrot mouth
- Class two malocclusion
- Overjet
- Mandibular brachygnathism

An overbite malocclusion is never considered normal in any breed and is a genetic fault. Most commonly affected breeds are those with elongated muzzles (collies, shelties, dachshunds, and Russian wolfhounds). If the mandibular canines or incisors penetrate the maxilla, crown reduction via vital pulpotomy or orthodontic tooth movement are two options.

An **underbite** occurs when the mandibular teeth protrude in front of the maxillary teeth (Fig. 7.112). This may lead to the maxillary incisors causing ulcers on the mandible. If ulceration is present, crown reduction via vital pulpotomy or extraction is indicated. (Figures 7.113–7.117 depict crown reduction and vital pulpotomy to treat a feline underbite.) Some short muzzled breeds normally have an underbite. If it occurs in a medium or long muzzled breed, it is abnormal. An underbite malocclusion is also commonly called

- Undershot
- Prognathism
- Class three malocclusion

When the maxillary and mandibular incisor teeth meet each other edge to edge, the occlusion is an even, or **level**, bite (Fig. 7.118). A level bite causes increased contact between maxillary and mandibular incisors, which can cause uneven wear, periodontal disease, and early tooth loss. A level bite is considered normal in some breeds although it is an expression of an underbite.

An **anterior crossbite** occurs when the canine and premolar teeth on both sides of the mouth occlude normally but one or more of the mandibular incisors are positioned in front of the maxillary incisors. This condition is caused by tug-of-war games, retained primary teeth, skeletal malocclusion, or impacted roots. An anterior crossbite, the most common malocclusion, is not considered genetic, unless there are skeletal growth problems. Treatment entails orthodontic movement of the abnormally positioned teeth by elastics attached to a labial arch bar (Figs 7.119 and 7.120).

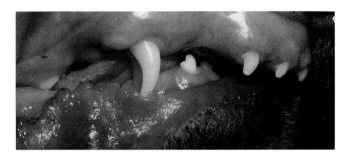

Fig. 7.111. Overbite malocclusion.

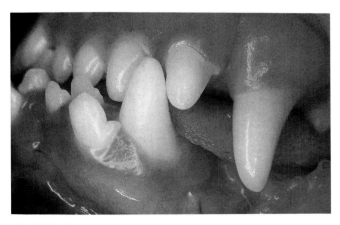

Fig. 7.112. Underbite malocclusion. Note mandibular canine rostral to lateral incisor.

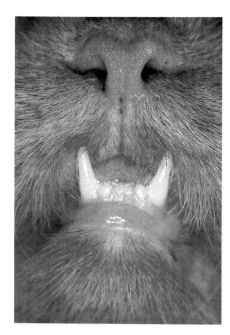

Fig. 7.113. Underbite in cat causing the mandibular canines and incisors to protrude rostral to the maxilla.

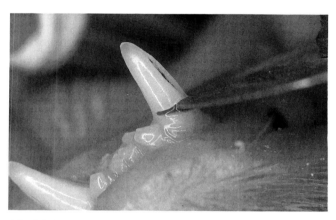

Fig. 7.114. Diamond disk used to reduce crown height of mandibular canines.

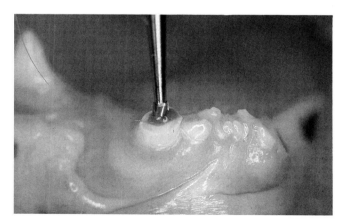

Fig. 7.115. Crown reduction and vital pulpotomy of mandibular canines.

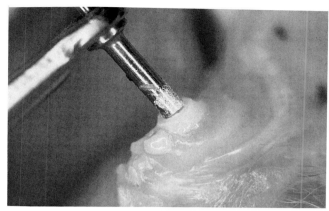

Fig. 7.116. Application of calcium hydroxide in vital pulpotomy procedure.

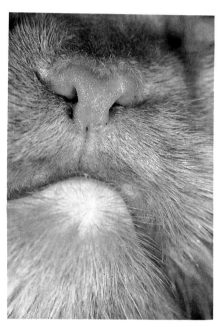

Fig. 7.117. Postoperatively, cat's lips can extend over mandible.

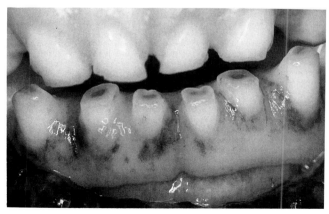

Fig. 7.118. Level bite.

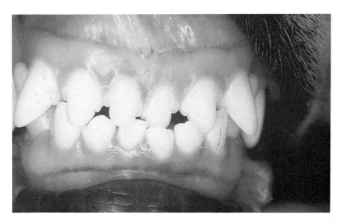

Fig. 7.119. Anterior crossbite.

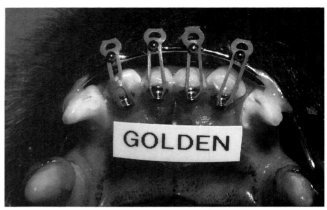

Fig. 7.120. Arch wire, brackets, and elastics used to correct anterior crossbite.

If there is an anterior crossbite, there must be a condition termed **posterior crossbite** (7.121). Posterior crossbite occurs when one or more of the premolar mandibular teeth buccally occlude with the maxillary teeth. This is a rare, inherited condition without treatment that occurs in the longer muzzled dog breeds, especially collies.

A **wry bite**, or wry mouth, occurs when one side of the jaw grows more than the other (Fig. 7.122). It is considered an inherited defect. A triangular defect where the teeth do not meet is noted in the incisor area.

Base narrow canines occur when the mandibular canine teeth protrude inward and penetrate the maxillary palate. This condition is due to retained deciduous teeth or from a too narrow mandible compared with the maxilla. Base narrow canines may be corrected either through orthodontic devices applied to the maxillary canine teeth used to push mandibular canine teeth laterally or through mandibular canine crown reduction (Figs. 7.123–7.126).

An **open bite** is seen in the incisor area often in conjunction with a wry bite. Affected teeth are displaced vertically and do not touch.

Rotated teeth, especially the maxillary third and fourth premolars, occur often in short muzzled breeds. In these dogs, selective breeding created an undersized mouth that cannot accommodate 42 teeth in normal alignment. The rotated tooth root closest to the palate is prone to bone loss and periodontal disease. Strict toothbrushing may be helpful in saving a rotated tooth. Often the tooth is extracted.

Rostral displacement of the upper or lower canine teeth, also referred to as **mesioversion**, may be caused by retained deciduous teeth or skeletal abnormalities. In the feline this rostral displacement is commonly called a "lance" or "spear" tooth. Persians are commonly affected.

Treatment of mesioversion involves either crown reduction and vital pulpotomy of the offending tooth or orthodontic movement with elastics (Figs. 7.127–7.129).

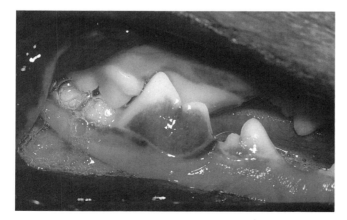

Fig. 7.121. Posterior crossbite.

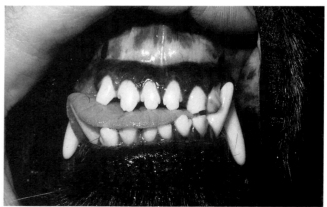

Fig. 7.122. Wry bite.

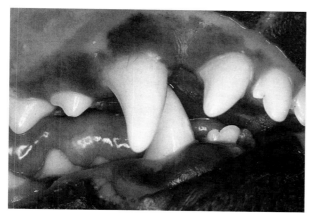

Fig. 7.123. *Base narrow canines. Notice mandibular canine penetrating maxilla.*

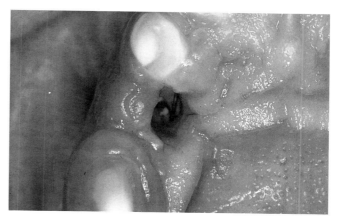

Fig. 7.124. *Penetration into hard palate by base narrow canine.*

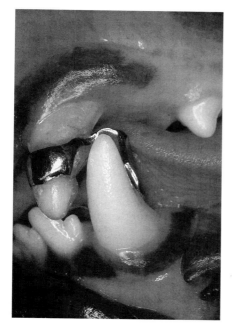

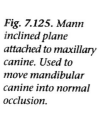

Fig. 7.125. *Mann inclined plane attached to maxillary canine. Used to move mandibular canine into normal occlusion.*

Fig. 7.126. *Acrylic inclined plane used to redirect mandibular canines to correct base narrow canines.*

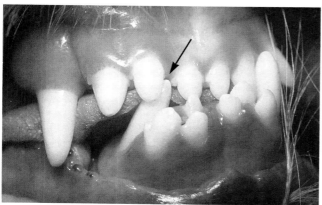

Fig. 7.127. *Rostral deviation of mandibular canine (arrow).*

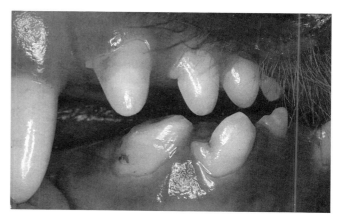

Fig. 7.128. *Crown reduction and vital pulpotomy removing contact.*

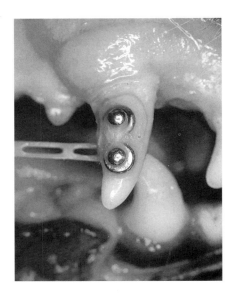

The anchor point for the elastic is the upper fourth premolar and/or the mandibular first molar. An elastic with 2 to 6 oz of tension is stretched between the canine and anchor teeth to gently pull the canine into normal occlusion. The elastic is changed weekly.

Fig. 7.129. Elastics and brackets used to correct rostral canine displacement.

❧Orthodontic Care at a Glance

Problem	Appearance	Treatment
Retained deciduous teeth	Two teeth in the same socket at the same time	Retained deciduous tooth extracted
Dental interlock	When the mandibular canines or incisors are impeding the forward growth of the maxilla	Interceptive orthodontics performed to remove the deciduous teeth interfering with maxillary forward growth
Extra teeth	Normally there are six maxillary and six mandibular incisors in the dog and cat. Look for extra incisors or premolars.	Extraction if overcrowding results
Overbite occlusion	Look for mandibular canines penetrating the hard palate.	Either crown reduction and vital pulpotomy of mandibular canines or orthodontic movement
Underbite occlusion	Look for mandibular penetration by maxillary incisors.	Crown reduction and vital pulpotomy if mandibular penetrations are ulcerated
Anterior crossbite	One or more mandibular incisors rostral to maxillary incisors	Orthodontic correction with arch wire and elastics
Base narrow canines	Mandibular canines penetrating into hard palate	Mandibular crown reduction or inclined plane attached to maxillary canines to push mandibular canines into normal occlusion
Rotated third premolars	Examine for crowding or periodontal pocket on palatal side of rotated tooth.	Extraction if pathology noted
Rostral displacement of upper or lower canines	Canines will be angled rostrally and may interfere with other teeth.	Crown reduction and vital pulpotomy or orthodontic movement with elastics

ANTIMICROBIAL USE IN DENTISTRY

For humans the American Dental Association recommends the use of antibiotics any time blood is present during an oral procedure. Three decisions about antimicrobial agents must be made with each dental procedure.

- When to prescribe antibiotics
- Which one to choose
- How long to use antimicrobials

When to Prescribe Antibiotics

Normally, there is a protective barrier between the oral cavity and the blood system. When this barrier is compromised, antibiotics are used to protect the patient. This barrier may be compromised due to

- Poor nutrition
- Concurrent heart or kidney failure
- Steroid medication
- A preexisting debilitating disease
- Metallic implants that may be seeded by bacteremia
- Cases of advanced periodontal disease
- Cases of osteomyelitis
- Ulcerative stomatitis
- Tooth fracture with pulpal exposure
- Gingivitis and periodontal disease
- Laceration of the oral mucosa

What Type of Antibiotics to Use

It is difficult to choose antibiotics based on patient presentation. From visual examination what may appear as grade two gingivitis may have some areas of bone loss secondary to periodontal disease. What may appear from the outside to be a normal patient may actually be one who harbors undiagnosed lesions necessitating periodontal pathogen-sensitive antibiotics.

It is best to use an antibiotic that will take care of most oral infections. Such an antibiotic must

- Be quickly delivered to the site of infection—preferably by white blood cells
- Cover a broad spectrum of bacteria, both aerobic and anaerobic
- Penetrate bone
- Be approved for use in dental infections

Different Antibiotic Regimens

- Give orally two days before dental procedure, then by injection pre- and postoperatively.

- Give orally preoperatively (clindamycin achieves effective blood levels within 20 minutes).

- Give by injection one hour before dental procedure.

- Give postoperatively for various lengths of time, depending on degree of infection. Minimum time given should be one week.

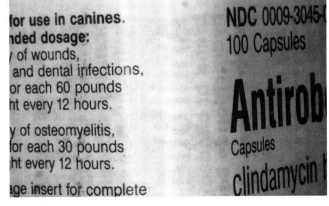

Fig. 7.130. Antirobe (Pharmacia & Upjohn Animal Health) is an antibiotic specifically indicated to treat dental infections.

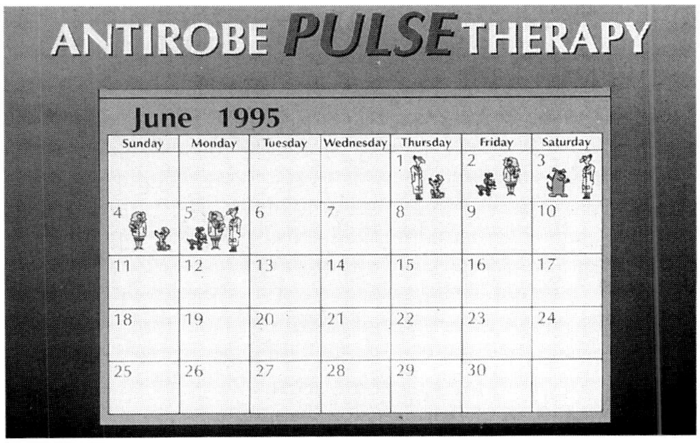

Fig. 7.131.

• When used as pulse therapy, give first five days of each month to help control periodontal disease. Advantages of pulse therapy include

— Decreases plaque production and adherence to dental structures
— Decreases bacterial load subgingivally
— Decreases halitosis
— Decreases growth of periodontal pathogens
— If given at label dosage, should not induce resistant strains because resistance occurs from using too much or too little of a dose for an increased length of time (weeks or months). Resistance also occurs in a stepwise fashion. Because pulse therapy is only given for five days, the resistance does not occur.

PAIN CONTROL MEDICATION

Animals feel pain like we do. When any dental procedure is performed that could be associated with patient discomfort, medication must be used to decrease pain. Dental procedures commonly associated with pain include

• Extractions
• Periodontal surgery
• Deep cleaning and root planing
• Subgingival curettage
• Root canal therapy
• Endodontics
• Oral surgery

8. PROPOSING CARE

The important thing in life is to have a great aim and to possess the aptitude and the perseverance to attain it.
—JOHANN WOLFGANG VON GOETHE

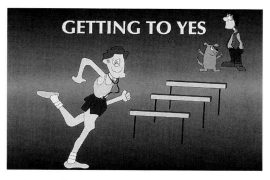

Fig. 8.1.

The best veterinary diagnosticians or surgeons will not get the opportunity to practice their dental talents without client permission. Helping you to determine what goes on inside your client's mind and identifying the best way to get the client to accept your dental recommendations are the goals of this chapter.

You need to convince your client that dental pathology is present and immediate therapy is necessary. Not only do you have to explain that a pet needs dental care you also have to find ways to make sure your client understands

- Why therapy has to be done now

  — Most dental pathology is progressive and, if not treated, may become untreatable.
  — If not now, then when? As soon as they leave the office, many clients forget the importance of the treatment as well as the disease.

- Fees and payment arrangements
- What the client will have to do for home care

Sounds like a tall order? Not if you cut it up into small, bite-sized pieces that make the proposed care digestible.

CASE PRESENTATION—SEEING IS BELIEVING

How often during a physical examination have you noticed inflammation, swelling, and calculus at the gingival margins consistent with grade two or three periodontal disease? What do you do? Does that voice in back of your head start rationalizing that it's only a little inflammation and the patient is in for a skin problem anyway, or are you convinced that your patient really needs prompt dental care? Untreated gingivitis often progresses to supporting bone destruction, possible tooth mobility, and a myriad of internal medical ailments. Remember, *all periodontitis starts with gingivitis.* If you advise your clients to bring their pets back for treatment, some will, but many will not.

What happens to these consumers? Do the pet owners understand that bacteria are reproducing below the gingiva, producing by-products that in time may cause liver and kidney problems as well as destroy their pets' periodontia? They do not see the inflammation because their pets' lips cover the disease. (Out of sight, out of mind.) When a client shares your recommended dental treatment plan with the rest of the family, the reply often is "Why? Rover is eating great," and Rover's gingivitis continues to progress untreated.

Most owners care deeply for their pets and want existing problems treated. How do you get them involved in dentistry? How can they better appreciate the gravity of a condition and potential complications from noncompliance? Through the use of instant photography, dental models (Fig. 8.2), videos, and charts. Let clients *see* their pets' oral problems as if they were sitting on the nose of the dog or cat. Clients can see pathology more easily in pictures than in an animal's poorly illuminated oral cavity.

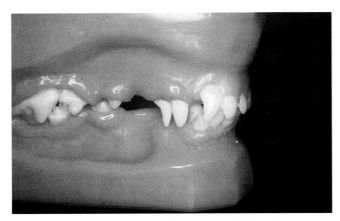

Fig. 8.2. Henry Schein dental model showing retained deciduous teeth.

Document the Oral Problem

During your physical examination, look at each tooth and show your client (if the dog or cat will allow) lesions or bite abnormalities. Be critical—any amount of gingival inflammation is abnormal and must be treated immediately. If the pet is in for a nondental problem (most are), still examine and note dental abnormalities.

Take a close-up Polaroid picture of any dog or cat with dental pathology. Even minor cases of gingivitis will show plaque and hyperemia at the gingival margin. Once the picture develops, let the pet owner compare it with a textbook representation of the disease. This confirms the pet's lesion is a real problem that needs care.

The picture will

- Allow your client to see oral pathology without having the pet's mouth handled for prolonged periods

- Permanently document pathology you noted in your exam. The picture should be enlarged to allow the veterinarian, staff, and client to see lesions better.

- Provide a take-home view of pathology your client can show family members

- Be a reminder, when posted in a prominent location at home (a refrigerator door or bathroom mirror), for the client either to return the pet to the office for dental care or to provide daily home care

- Provide your client with before and after photographs. These serve as accurate, readily comprehensible, and visually impacting documentation

of your skills. Leave one set in the medical record and give one to your client to show those at home.

- Enable you to send before and after pictures to referral veterinarians

- Provide a pictorial history of a patient's oral lesions

- Become part of a bulletin board or smile book, which displays pictures before and after treatment, to show other clients and staff the dental cases you have handled (Fig. 8.3)

- Create a teaching file so that new staff can get acquainted with oral pathology and treatment possibilities

- Memorialize cases for future study or reference

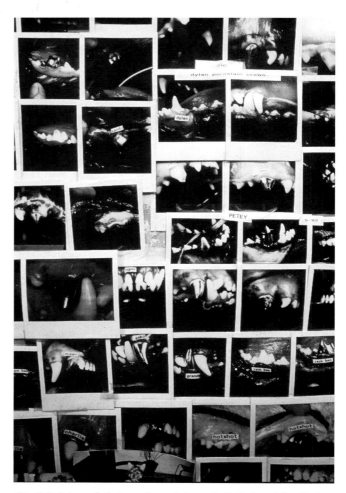

Fig. 8.3. Intraoral photographs posted on a bulletin board for clients to see.

35-MM PHOTOGRAPHY

With new technology, cameras and their flashes now have a symbiotic relationship—they electronically communicate with each other to obtain optimum results. The flash comes in point source or ring choices. The ring light is a circular flash tube. It will produce shadow-free, uniform illumination by flooding the subject with light from all angles. The "point flash" choice will create a picture with highlighted areas.

Slide images can be stored according to discipline in plastic holders in notebooks. (For instance all endodontic cases in one notebook; all periodontal cases in another.)

The camera system we use is the Lester A. Dine Auto Exposure System. The system includes a 35-mm camera, a 100-mm macro lens, a 1:1 auto converter, and a dedicated flash with both ring and point capabilities. We set the camera on automatic and use the through-the-lens focusing capability to get perfect exposures.

Some helpful "add-ons" when choosing a camera include a motorized drive and data back (to stamp the date on pictures).

INTRAORAL INSTANT PHOTOGRAPHY

The instant picture gives the client an immediate picture of pathology. Intraoral instant cameras are available through Lester A. Dine, Inc., in Palm Beach Gardens, Florida (800-624-9103). There are two popular models to choose from.

- The Macro 5 SLRV ($800), which has five built-in enlargement options (Fig. 8.4)

- The Dine Instant Veterinary Close-up Kit model A1V ($400), which comes with attachable close-up lenses (Figs 8.5 and 8.6)

The **MedRx instant video system** produces single or multiple instant photos captured from a monitor screen (Fig. 8.7). Split photos of before and after views of dental pathology help to educate pet owners on the severity of disease present and how it resolved following care. Multiple instant-picture copies of the frozen video screen can be made for your client, smile book, bulletin board, and patient chart.

SLIDE DUPLICATOR

We use a Polaroid slide duplicator that produces enlarged, instant pictures to show clients and referring veterinarians close-ups of dental radiographs (Fig. 8.8). For radiograph copy, the nonscreened film is placed in a slide holder and inserted into the slide duplicator. A 3× enlargement is delivered about one minute later.

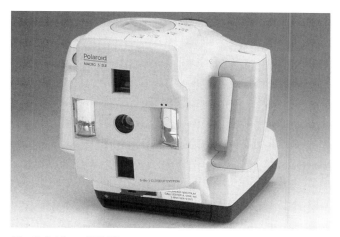

Fig. 8.4. Macro 5 SLRV camera.

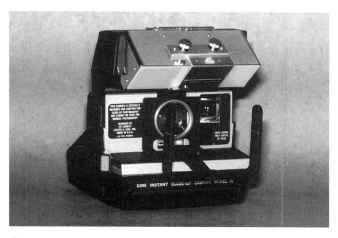

Fig. 8.5. Lester A. Dine Instant Veterinary Close-up Polaroid camera.

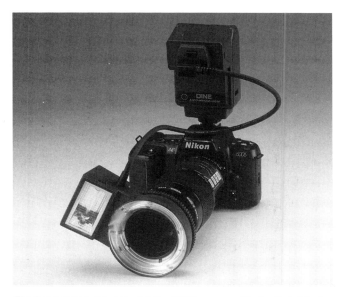

Fig. 8.6. Lester A. Dine Dental Eye SLRV camera with ring/point flash.

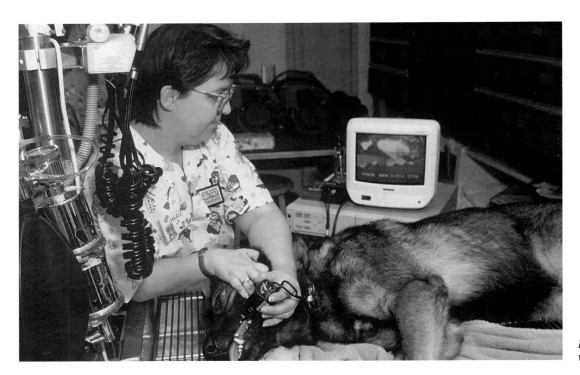

Fig. 8.7. MedRx videoscope system.

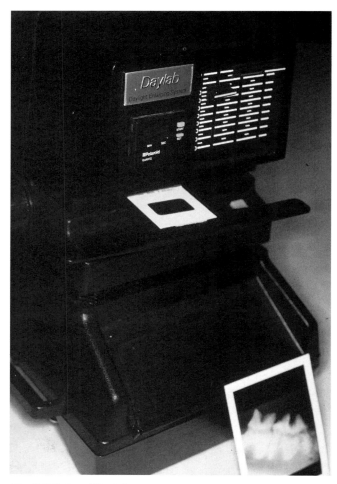

Fig. 8.8. Polaroid Daylab.

Convince Your Client to Act

This is the time to educate clients about the benefits of dental care. With therapy your patients will usually

- Live in less pain
- Be healthier
- Live longer
- Smell better
- Eat better

Review the Procedure Used

Tell your client what you plan to do from the beginning to the end. Don't just say, "We are going to clean Fifi's teeth today." Review the 12 steps of the professional teeth-cleaning visit. Be sure to include in your description:

- Preoperative testing
- Anesthesia—how it is delivered and safety precautions
- A description of actual surgery, if applicable. Use a smile book, which depicts the steps. People understand pictures better than words.
- How you manage pet pain
- Postoperative care to be given by the owner

OVERCOMING OBJECTIONS

There are four main objections made by clients when asked to allow pet dental procedures: the perceived danger of anesthesia, the cost of procedures, postoperative pain, and the inability to perform home care.

Anesthesia

The client's most significant objection to dental procedures is anesthesia. Many clients know of an animal that died at a veterinarian's office while under anesthesia. This is a concern that needs to be discussed. Often clients let their pets suffer needlessly with severe periodontal disease rather than risk anesthesia. Unfortunately, far more pets die unnecessarily from complications of periodontal disease than from anesthesia.

You must instill confidence that anesthetics are safely administered in your office. This can be done by explaining that you

- Prescreen patients with laboratory testing. Depending on an animal's age and condition, tests include blood, urine, and stool, an electrocardiogram, and chest radiographs.

- Use the safest anesthetic and deliver it in the safest manner. To help with safety,

  — Place intravenous catheters in pets prior to induction.
  — Intubate all dental cases and maintain with inhalant anesthetics.

- Monitor all anesthesia patients. Use appearance of the gingiva, electrocardiograph, pulse oximetry, blood pressure, and end tidal carbon dioxide monitoring.

Cost

Cost is a client concern. Don't bring this up until the end of your discussion, after your client is convinced his or her pet needs the procedure. When fees are discussed early, your client begins to think about the money and stops listening to the whys, whats, and hows. Let your client understand your diagnosis, the need for therapy, and the consequences if therapy is not done. Then ask if the client can leave the pet for treatment. The client will either say yes or no depending on his or her schedule. Before the client leaves your office, discuss fees.

If your client understands that the procedure needs to be done, wants to let you proceed, but does not have the funds for therapy, there are options (see "Financial Arrangements").

Postoperative Pain

Your ability to control the pet's pain is the basis of much of the owner's anxiety. People equate dental procedures with pain. Fortunately, it is easy and inexpensive to control pain with medication. All animals undergoing any type of painful procedure must be given medication to control their discomfort.

Inability to Provide Home Care

Inability to provide home care is a concern due to lack of client education. You must have a staff member in charge of reviewing instructions with your client and demonstrating how to take care of the pet's teeth to ensure future oral health. After the exit interview, your client must not be forgotten. Follow-up appointments should be made first weekly then monthly to see how effectively your client is providing home care.

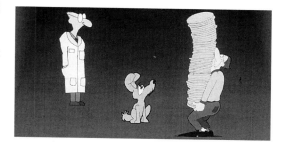

Fig. 8.9.

DENTAL FEE SHEETS

When your patient presents with an involved orthopedic, dermatological, or intestinal problem, there are separate fees for examination, diagnostics, therapy, and "take home" medication. Why not the same for dental care?

The only way to approach a dental case is to address each tooth or oral problem individually. If a patient presented with a femoral fracture and an elbow luxation, fees for care would be itemized separately. Lumping the care of all oral conditions under "doing a dentistry" and charging one set fee is poor business, and not providing individual tooth care is poor medicine.

Evaluating each tooth on its own merit and itemizing fees relating to individual tooth care is a rational way to approach dental case management. An itemized fee sheet will help you organize your thoughts into an orderly treatment plan. Your client will readily appreciate fees related to dental care when they are presented in a printed format.

How to Create a Dental Fee Sheet

Fees are related to the expense of providing care. Each practice performs a different level of dental care. Some practitioners provide advanced endodontic, periodontal, and orthodontic therapy, while others examine, clean, polish, and extract mobile or fractured teeth.

The services provided should be listed on the dental fee sheet in a logical order. Begin with **examination** and **preoperative diagnostics** (determined by age or physical condition). **Anesthesia** is covered as a separate listing. Preanesthesia medication costs the practice and is itemized separately. For general anesthesia some practices charge flat fees while others charge by the minute or hour. Supervising patient response to anesthesia with pulse oximetry, blood pressure, electrocardiogram, or respiratory monitoring is expensive for the practice and is itemized as an hourly expense.

Radiology is an important aspect of dental diagnostics. Intraoral radiographs help the practitioner determine if a tooth can be saved or should be extracted. Some veterinarians list a standard fixed radiology fee; others charge per film.

A complete list of **dental services** follows on the fee sheet, beginning with teeth cleaning. Differentiate cleaning fees based on the degree of disease present. Care for advanced periodontal disease is more involved than that for gingivitis and is listed separately. Enter this data into your computer system so that itemizing by degree of periodontal disease automatically triggers checkup reminders at intervals that are tied into the degree of pathology.

Extraction fees can be tabulated by the number of roots involved. A triple-rooted tooth usually takes more expertise, equipment, and time to extract: its extraction should cost more than the removal of a single-rooted tooth. Some practitioners itemize extractions based on the amount of mobility of the tooth, degree of difficulty involved, or time spent on the procedure. (I don't agree with this method because the more efficiently you practice, and the greater your expertise, the less you get paid.)

Periodontal therapy may be itemized to include root planing, curettage, fluoride treatment, apical reposition surgery, and guided tissue regeneration. Many practitioners base endodontic care on the number of roots treated. The components of crown preparation, impression, repeat anesthesia, and cementation are included on the fee sheet. Additionally, fees for orthodontic stone models, laboratory work, and bracket placement should be listed separately.

Antibiotics, **analgesic medication**, and **oral hygiene supplies** are also itemized. Home care is the foundation of long-term dental success.

How to Use the Dental Fee Sheet

After the client is made aware of the pet's dental problems and the treatment plan, he or she will usually ask about fees. Use your fee list as a worksheet. Circle those procedures relating to the treatment plan. Present the ideal treatment plan first. Then escort the client to the receptionist, who will total the fee sheet, collect a prepayment, and admit the patient for treatment.

Most times, an exact treatment plan fee cannot be determined when your client is in the exam room because, to evaluate each tooth, the patient must be examined under anesthesia, with radiographs taken. Give your client a partially circled fee sheet with procedures you plan to perform in order to make a diagnosis (preoperative testing, administration of anesthetics, insertion of an intravenous catheter, radiographs, teeth cleaning). Your client should take the fee sheet home so that he or she has it when calling at a predetermined time to find out

- What your exam findings are—the diagnosis
- What you can do to treat the pathology
- What the fees are
- When the client can pick up the dog or cat

Setting Fees

Expenses are related to costs. Each practice's fees are different in that expenses differ. The fee sheet in Figure 8.10 is a list of our practice's fees based on our expenses. Your dental fee sheet will be different. *Charge what you need to in order to provide ideal dental care for your clients.* Fees must include the cost of equipment, additional staff, and those expenses you incurred obtaining your dental education.

If you educate them, clients commonly accept fees similar to what they pay for their own dentistry. Take the time to explain how your procedures are the same as their dentists' and that veterinary dentistry requires similar instruments and knowledge.

Win, Win, Win

Thanks to word processors and printers, preparing a fee sheet is an easy job. It is simple to change entries, based on your expertise and client feedback. Everyone wins when you use a dental fee sheet: the practice benefits through greater productivity, you practice dentistry in a more organized manner, and most importantly the patient benefits from logical, orderly care.

Eighty-five percent of all dogs and cats have dental disease that needs immediate care. If you are not introducing

ALL PETS DENTAL CLINIC

Dental Consultation	Exam	$ 65.00	DEX
Preoperative Testing	Complete Blood Count	28.25	CBC
<1 YR CBC	Kidney Function Test	27.25	KFT
1–4 YRS CBC, Total Protein	Liver Function Test	22.25	LFT
4–7 YRS CBC, Liver, Kidney	Total Protein Test	24.25	TPT
> 7 YRS CBC, Organ Profile	Blood Sugar Test	21.25	BST
Electrolytes, Urine, EKG	Organ Profile	71.25	CPT
	Electrolytes	36.25	ELEC
	Complete Urinalysis	24.75	UAC
	EKG	55.25	CECG
	Intravenous Catheter	22.00	SETIV
	Intravenous Fluids	20.00	FLUID
Preanesthetic Sedation		28.00	MSED
Loacal Anesthesia (Per Quadrant)		29.00	LOCAL
Anesthesia Per Hour		71.00	ANES
Pulse Oximeter Per Hour		15.00	POX
Dental Radiographs	One to Three Views	40.00	DRAD
	Each Additional View	9.95	DRADA
Cleaning and Polishing	Gingivitis	45.00	DCPG
	Advanced Gingivitis	55.00	DCPGA
	Periodontics	70.00	DCPP
	Fluoride Treatment	12.00	DFL
Endodontics	Single-Rooted Tooth	200.00	DEND1
	Double-Rooted Tooth	250.00	DEND2
	Triple-Rooted Tooth	300.00	DEND3
	Surgical Endondontics–Apicoectomy	350.00	DENDS
Extractions	Single-Rooted Tooth (first premolar, incisor)	54.00	DEXT1
	Double-Rooted Tooth	75.00	DEXT2
	Triple-Rooted Tooth	115.00	DEXT3
	Canine	125.00	DEXTC
	Deciduous Tooth	54.00	DEXTD
Crowns	Rubber Impressions	95.00	DCRI
	Crown Prep	75.00	DCP
	Lab Fees	200.00	DCLF
	Crown Cementation	40.00	DCC
	Repeat Anesthesia and Pulse Oximeter	86.00	DCRA
Periodontics	Flap Surgery (per quadrant)	125.00	DPFS
	Root Planing	25.00	DPRS
	Gingivectomy	60.00	DPG
	Guided Tissue Regeneration	125.00	DPGTR
Restorative Care	Cat Neck Lesion–Glass Ionomer	60.00	DRNL
	Bonding	40.00	DRB
Orthodontics	Stone Studey Models	125.00	DOSS
	Orthodontic Care	750.00	DOC
	Lab Fees	525.00	DOLF
Antibiotic Injection		18.00	IANT
Discomfort Injection		18.00	IP
Hospitalization	Per Night	35.00	HOSP
Home Care	Oral–Gel	12.95	ORALG
	CET Finger Brush	3.99	FBR
	Finger Brush Kit	6.95	FDK
	CET Toothpaste	6.95	CET
	CET Spray	6.95	CETS
	CET Spray w/Fluoride	7.95	CETS
	CET Chews	5.95	CETG

Fig. 8.10. Dental fee sheet.

the need for pet dental services to 8 or 9 of every 10 clients who walk through your door, you are missing benefits to your patient, client, and practice.

FINANCIAL ARRANGEMENTS

When the doctor and/or any member of the staff act as if payment is not important, the patient will also believe this is true. We do not want to aggressively demand full payment from each client; however, a veterinary practice cannot continue to see patients when fees are not collected.

Often your client cannot (or does not want to) afford fees related to care. You have established the need for service, but your client may consider not having the care due to the expense. Most dental care is not planned for ahead of time and is not a budgeted family expense. Rather than having the pet suffer from dental neglect, there are payment options. Do not accept no for an answer when an animal needs dental care. There is a way to find yes, although it takes tenacity at times. Keep your patient's benefit foremost in your mind. Some helpful ways to get to yes:

- Offer credit card payment plans, which allow the patient to be treated and the practice to get paid through monthly payments. For example, offer a postdated credit card policy. Ask the owner to agree to your billing his or her credit card company monthly according to an agreed upon schedule.

- Medical charge companies (Dencharge, through the American Animal Hospital Association, and Medcash, 800-800-5759) will loan creditworthy clients the funds for therapy and allow them to pay as little as $30 monthly. Clients are usually accepted if they have a job that pays $1000 per month, good credit, and a checking account.

- Offer a held check policy, where half the fee is paid at the time of service, and the remaining fee is divided over a three- or six-month period. Checks should be predated (preferably with the date of deposit) and deposited on the first of every month.

SEVEN STEPS TO EDUCATE YOUR CLIENT ABOUT THE NEED FOR DENTAL CARE

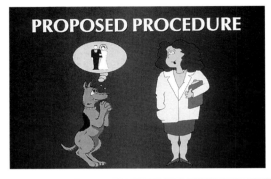

Fig. 8.11.

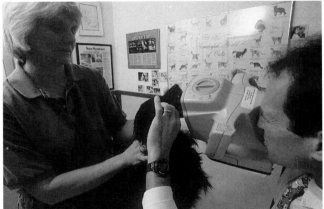

Fig. 8.12.

1 The first step is informing clients that their pets need care. You must show them there is a problem. Clients bring their pets to us because the animals have medical problems, are suffering from internal or external parasites, or need vaccinations, not because they have too many or missing teeth, inflamed gums, or bad breath. Most clients accept bad breath in their dogs or cats as natural.

Instant photographs are the most efficient way to document oral problems for clients. In a matter of seconds, enlarged photos can be developed that depict retained deciduous teeth, feline odontoclastic resorptions, fractured teeth, and gingival disease.

2 A dental model, alongside the intraoral picture, is a powerful tool for convincing clients that their pets need dental care (Fig. 8.13). For example, when a dog has a retained deciduous tooth, the mandibular portion of the model shows the retained tooth pushing the adult tooth aside. The maxillary part of the model shows what can happen with neglect—an inflamed opening into the nasal passage.

3 Use a smile book (Fig. 8.14). Dentistry is virgin territory for most clients. A book with before and after pictures will reinforce your recommendations that your proposed care will result in improved health.

4 Confirm the diagnosis and treatment plan with literature. Some clients will need more information before they commit to needed dental work. Collect articles on common dental problems. Start files on periodontics, endodontics, orthodontics, and oral surgery. Make sure the articles show pictures of the problem and cover therapy. Recommend the best therapy available. Only your client can decrease the level of care you give.

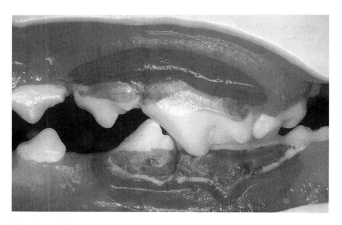

Fig. 8.13. *Pharmacia & Upjohn Animal Health dental model.*

5 Ask your clients to leave their pets. By this point in the consultation, you have demonstrated through photography, models, and literature why their pets need dental care. Ask if you can *borrow* their pets to treat the dental problems. Make recommendations as if they did not cost anything, and your clients will find a way to afford your services. They either can or cannot leave their pets. If your clients' schedules do not permit you to care for their pets immediately, give them instant pictures to remind them that their pets still have the problems that need therapy.

6 Once your clients have agreed to the dental procedures, discuss fees. The best way to do this is with a preprinted dental fee sheet with items circled in the exam room and totaled at the receptionist's desk. Your concern must not be centered on the fees but on the costs to the pet if a client does not agree to dental care.

7 Be firm with your recommendations. Remember that clients come to you for expert evaluation of their pets' health. Your firm conviction will reassure them they are making the right decision by leaving their pets for necessary dental care. When you send an animal home with untreated pathology, everyone loses.

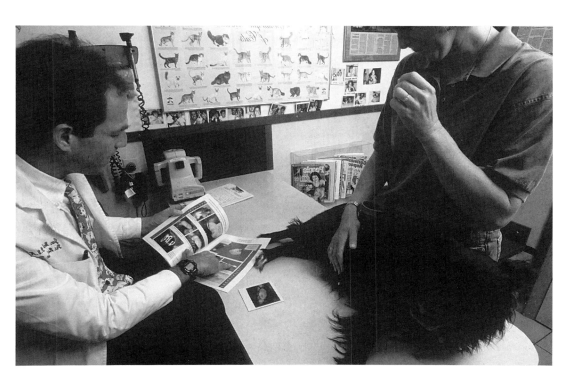

Fig. 8.14.
The Smile Book,
by author.

Appendix 1
❧CLIENT HANDOUTS AND OTHER DENTAL CARE FORMS

[Your letterhead here]

Frenquently Asked Dental Questions and Their Answers

Why should I brush my pet's teeth?

Daily removal of plaque is the key to an effective oral hygiene program. Unless your pet's teeth are brushed daily, plaque, which is an accumulation of bacteria, will build up at the gum line. Eventually, calculus forms, further irritating the gums, causing infection that progresses to destroy the attachment around your pet's teeth. In addition to creating loose teeth, infection under the gum line can spread to the liver, kidneys, and heart.

How can I brush my pet's teeth?

It is usually a very easy and fun procedure. First, pick a soft-bristled or finger toothbrush. Next, get toothpaste from your veterinarian. Do not use toothpaste intended for humans because it has detergents that should not be swallowed. Apply a small amount of toothpaste on the toothbrush and brush the outside of the upper cheek teeth. Concentrate on the area where the tooth meets the gum line.

How often does my pet need to have its teeth cleaned by the veterinarian?

It depends on the degree of plaque and tartar accumulation. Examine your pet's teeth monthly. Look for an accumulation of yellow or brown material at the area where the tooth meets the gum line. Pay particular attention to the cheek teeth and canines.

Once you notice plaque or tartar accumulation, it is time for a professional cleaning. Do not wait. Attached to the tartar are bacteria that are irritating gum tissues. When treated, inflammation will be resolved. When gingivitis is left untreated, it will progress to periodontitis, which is nonreversible.

The intervals between teeth-cleaning procedures will depend on how often you can brush your pet's teeth. Once or twice daily is optimum. If you cannot brush your pet's teeth, then your pet will probably need two or three professional teeth-cleaning visits yearly.

Can I just take my fingernail or a dental scaler to remove the calculus?

Dental disease occurs below the gum line. By removing calculus from the visible part of the tooth, you are not removing disease below the gum line. In order to help your pet, plaque and calculus must be removed from below the gum line.

Do you have to use anesthetics to clean my pet's teeth?

Anesthesia is necessary when performing teeth cleaning. Anesthesia provides three important functions: immobilization in order to clean below the gum line, pain control, and the ability to place a tube into the windpipe so bacterial products do not enter the respiratory system.

I am concerned about the anesthesia. Is it safe?

We take every effort to ensure anesthetics are safely administered. We use the safest of anesthetic agents. All dogs and cats are given preoperative tests, depending on their age and condition, to qualify them as candidates for anesthesia. Finally, while anesthetized, all animals are monitored with electrocardiogram oscilloscopes, blood pressure monitors, and pulse oximeters.

What is involved in the teeth cleaning at your hospital?

For each professional teeth cleaning, 12 separate procedures are performed:

1. A general exam before anesthesia, including evaluation of the bite, preoperative organ testing, and identification of abnormal wear patterns, gum infection, and oral cancer
2. Oral examination of each tooth under anesthesia
3. Calculus removal from the visible part of the teeth
4. Subgingival (below-the-gum-line) scaling, root planing, and curettage where indicated

5. Tooth polishing
6. Irrigation
7. Fluoride application
8. A postcleaning exam and radiographs if needed
9. Dental charting to keep a record of abnormalities
10. Therapy if necessary
11. Home care instructions
12. A no fee follow-up appointment and periodic rechecks to see how well you are performing home care

How much does a tooth-cleaning procedure cost?

It is impossible to quote what the procedure will cost because we do not know what state your pet's teeth and gums are in. There are four levels of teeth cleanings at our hospital. The range of fees is based on severity plus fees for preoperative testing, anesthesia, necessary therapy, and medication. The doctor or staff will be happy to give you an estimate once you bring your dog or cat in for the examination.

What is best to feed my pet?

Hard food will help remove plaque from teeth. There are special diets specifically manufactured to help keep dogs' and cats' teeth clean. Feeding these special diets in conjunction with daily brushing is the best way to keep the teeth clean. Diet alone will not control plaque, but it will help.

What toys should I avoid to protect my pet's teeth?

Chewing on objects harder than the tooth may lead to dental fractures. Be especially careful with cow and horse hooves. They commonly cause fractures of the upper cheek teeth. Do not play tug-of-war games, especially with young dogs and cats, because they can move growing teeth to abnormal locations. Throwing dogs Frisbees can also cause trauma to the teeth resulting in pulpitis (an inflammation of the pulp).

What are cat cavities?

Many cats get painful lesions at the gum line that invade the teeth. The lesions are referred to as feline odontoclastic resorptive lesions (FORLs). Unfortunately, we do not know what causes FORLs, and the most effective treatment involves extraction of the affected tooth. Check to see if your cat has a FORL by placing a cotton-tipped applicator to the gum line and pressing. If there is a painful lesion, your cat will chatter its jaw and must be treated.

How can I tell if my pet is suffering from periodontal disease?

The leading sign is bad breath. Dogs and cats should not have disagreeable mouth odor. Bad breath comes from infection. If your pet's breath does not *smell like roses,* let us examine its mouth and advise care.

What types of tests are done to diagnose dental disease?

If periodontal disease is present or if your pet has a fractured tooth, an oral exam is performed while the pet is under anesthesia. A periodontal probe is used to evaluate bone loss around each tooth. Radiographs are taken to evaluate if teeth can be saved or need to be extracted.

When do I have to start worrying about dental problems with my pet?

As soon as puppy or kitten teeth emerge, it's time to start brushing. Although baby teeth are replaced with adult teeth, the puppy or kitten gets used to the brushing procedure, which continues for life.

What can be done if my pet has periodontal disease?

Periodontal disease occurs when tooth support structures are affected by infection. In the beginning stages, cleaning above and below the gum line as well as removal of calculus attached to the tooth will help restore periodontal health. In advanced cases, either periodontal surgery or extractions are performed. Antibiotics given monthly also help to control the progression of periodontal disease.

Which animals are at most risk for periodontal disease?

Smaller breeds are more prone than larger because the teeth are closer together in small dogs, and these dogs usually live longer. Terriers, Maltese, and Shih Tzus are especially prone to periodontal disease.

What can you do to fix a broken tooth?

If your dog or cat breaks its tooth, there are two treatments: root canal therapy to save the tooth or extraction. Leaving the tooth alone with an exposed nerve is not a humane option. In addition to pain, infection will develop, which can spread to vital organs.

[Your letterhead here]

Could My Dog or Cat Have Periodontal Disease?

Teeth are anchored in periodontal tissues consisting of gingiva (gums), ligaments, cementum, and supporting bone. More than 85 percent of dogs and cats older than four years have periodontal disease.

Periodontal disease starts with the formation of plaque, a transparent adhesive fluid composed of bacteria. Plaque starts forming within twelve hours after a thorough dental cleaning. When plaque is not removed, mineral salts in saliva hasten the formation of hard calculus. Calculus, covered with bacteria, is irritating to gingival tissue. By-products of bacteria "eat away" tooth support structures, causing pain and periodontal disease.

The mobility index evaluates tooth movement within the socket. With **class one** mobility, the tooth moves only slightly. **Class two** describes tooth movement less than the distance of a crown width. **Class three** mobility occurs when there is movement greater than a crown width. Class three reflects severe periodontal disease in which the teeth have lost more than 50 percent of their support and usually need extraction.

Periodontal disease can also be graded from stages one to four. The first two stages are classified as gingivitis; the last two as periodontitis. In **stage one**, plaque extends to the gum line, causing inflammation of the gingiva. **Stage two** gingivitis is marked by inflammation and swelling. Thorough teeth cleaning under anesthesia, followed by home care, can usually reverse gingivitis. If treated early, the gingiva can return to normal appearance and function. If untreated, periodontitis can result. **Stage three** periodontal disease occurs when there is bone loss in addition to gingival inflammation and infection. In **stage four** periodontal disease, there is progression of bone loss, usually creating tooth mobility.

Once bone loss from periodontal disease has occurred, more involved therapy than teeth cleaning is needed. What factors are considered before periodontal surgery? A cooperative patient, a treatable tooth, and a choice of which periodontal procedure to use.

The owner of a dog or cat with periodontal disease needs to be committed to saving the animal's teeth. This commitment includes daily brushing to remove plaque. Frequent veterinary dental reexaminations are also required, and expense should be considered.

The patient must also be a willing partner. If a dog or cat will not allow home care, the best dental surgeon and most caring owner will not make a difference. Unless there is strong owner commitment and patient compliance, it is wiser to extract a tooth rather than letting the pet suffer.

Choosing appropriate teeth to operate upon is equally important. Every dental procedure by a veterinarian should include probing and charting. The periodontal probe is an important instrument used to evaluate periodontal health. A probe is marked in millimeter gradations. It is gently inserted in the space between the gingival margin and tooth. The probe will stop where gingiva attaches to the tooth or at the bottom of the pocket if the attachment is gone. Dogs without periodontal disease should have less than 2-mm probing depths and cats less than 1. Each tooth must be probed on four sides. Probing depths of all teeth are noted on the pet's medical record, and a treatment plan formatted.

Pocket depths of up to 5 mm in both cats and dogs can usually be cleaned adequately with hand instruments and ultrasonic scaling. Depths greater than 5 mm need surgical care to clean the root surfaces or to extract the tooth.

Intraoral radiographs supply essential information for deciding which tooth will benefit from surgery. Radiographs help when evaluating supportive bone around the teeth. As a rule, if there is greater than 50 percent bone loss around a tooth, only advanced surgical procedures may provide long-term success.

Once the veterinarian is convinced that he or she is working on a cooperative patient and a tooth that can benefit from care, the appropriate type of periodontal surgery is chosen. An ideal method allows exposure of the root surface for cleaning, preserves attached gingiva, and allows gingiva to be reconnected in a fashion that eliminates the periodontal pocket.

[Your letterhead here; a handout on toothbrushing]

Brush My Dog's or Cat's What?

What would happen if you stopped brushing your own teeth? Even if you only ate hard food as some dogs and cats do, there still would be problems. Your pet's teeth must be brushed daily if you can manage it. It is not as difficult as you might imagine.

What are the benefits? Brushing removes the daily accumulation of plaque from the teeth. Although dogs and cats do not commonly get cavities, they do suffer from periodontal disease. If untreated, gum disease can lead to pain, infection of vital organs, and loss of teeth.

How to Brush Teeth

- **Step one**
  Pick an appropriate pet toothbrush.
  Save yourself time—do not buy a child's toothbrush with bristles too hard for small animals. The ideal dog toothbrush will have a long handle, an angled head to better fit the mouth, and extra-soft bristles. Cat toothbrushes are made with small handles and fine bristles to easily fit into smaller mouths. Finger toothbrushes are also available that fit over the tip of your finger.

- **Step two**
  Select the appropriate toothpaste.
  The best pet toothpastes contain enzymes that help control plaque. Avoid toothpastes with baking soda, detergents, or salt. Human toothpastes are not used because they are not made to be swallowed. Fluoride may be incorporated to help control bacteria. Rather than placing the paste on top of the brush, try to incorporate it between the bristles.

- **Step three**
  Get the brush with paste into your dog's or cat's mouth and begin brushing.
  Most pets accept brushing if they are approached in a gentle manner. If you start when they are young, it is quite easy, but even older pets will accept the process. Start slowly, using a washcloth or piece of gauze to wipe the teeth. Do this twice daily for about two weeks, and your pet will become familiar with the approach. Then take the pet toothbrush, soak it in warm water, and start brushing daily for several days. When your pet accepts this brushing, add the pet toothpaste.

- **Step four**
  The toothbrush bristles should be placed at a 45-degree angle at the gum margin, where the teeth and gums meet.
  Movement should be in an oval pattern. Be sure to gently place the bristle ends into the area around the base of the tooth as well as into spaces between teeth. Ten short back and forth motions are completed, and then the brush is moved to a new location. Cover three to four teeth at a time. Most attention should be given to the outside of the upper teeth.

How to Make the Toothbrushing Experience a Positive One

1. Choose an area of the house that is comfortable for you and your pet. Your pet should be lying on its side or sitting.

2. Start by handling the lips and gently rubbing the teeth with your fingers, without toothbrush or paste. If your dog or cat objects, stop and repeat later. Eventually extend the oral handling time (without a brush) from two to four minutes.

3. Rub the teeth with a piece of cheesecloth dipped in bouillon and wrapped around the index finger. Start with the front teeth, and as your pet becomes accustomed to the process, venture toward the cheek teeth.

4. Dogs like the taste of garlic. Unless your dog is in danger of having heart failure, dip a soft-bristled toothbrush into a solution of garlic salt and water. Let your dog lick the brush. Your pet will soon realize that

the toothbrush bristles taste good. Cats usually like the flavor of tuna fish. Dipping the toothbrush in the water from a tuna fish can will be helpful in getting your cat to accept oral hygiene.

5. When your pet is comfortable with this procedure, switch to a veterinary toothpaste and toothbrush. Do not use your toothpaste because it may cause vomiting due to detergents that should not be swallowed.

6. The toothbrush is placed at a 45-degree angle to the gum line. Bristles are placed at the gingival margin. A short back and forth or circular motion allowing the bristles to remain under the gingival margin is necessary to control plaque. Ten strokes in each area on the gum line is sufficient.

7. Concentrate brushing on the outside aspects of the teeth. The lingual and palatal surfaces are usually self-cleaned by the tongue.

8. Introducing the toothbrush is a process of building confidence and trust. Do not force your pet to accept it. Gentle encouragement works best. Be sure to reward progress.

[Your letterhead here; a handout to be given to breeders
on occlusion abnormalities]

Name That Bite ...

What is meant by the words *overbite, open bite, overjet, level bite, overshot, underbite, anterior crossbite, wry bite, retained deciduous teeth,* and *base narrow canines?* Breeders, show judges, veterinarians, and others who want to express specific dental conditions in dogs and cats need to use the proper terms. This article will review commonly used and misused words to describe tooth alignment.

Anatomy: Dogs normally have 28 deciduous (primary or baby) teeth that erupt during the first six months of life. Most breeds have 42 adult teeth. Cats have 26 deciduous and 30 adult teeth. There are four types of teeth. **Incisors** are the smaller teeth located between the canines on the upper and lower jaws. They are used for grasping food and help keep the tongue within the mouth. **Canines** (also called cuspids or fang teeth) are located on the sides of the incisors and used to grasp food. **Premolars** (bicuspids) are for shearing or cutting food and are located behind the canines. The **molars** are the last teeth to emerge in the mouth. They are used for grinding nourishment for entry into the esophagus.

Missing or Extra Teeth: Dogs and cats are frequently born without the proper number of teeth. Extra (supernumerary) teeth can cause periodontal disease from overcrowding. The American Kennel Club sets the standards concerning the minimum number of teeth for each breed of dog that can be shown. Dental radiographs can be safely taken as early as 10 weeks of age to evaluate if the correct number of adult teeth are present. This is recommended as a part of the prepurchase examination in certain breeds.

Occlusion: The way teeth align with each other is termed occlusion. Normal occlusion in most breeds consists of the upper (maxillary) incisors just overlapping the lower (mandibular) incisors (scissors bite). The lower canine should be located equidistant between the last (lateral) incisor and the upper canine tooth. Premolar tips of the lower jaw should point between the spaces of the upper jaw teeth. Flat-faced breeds (boxers, Shih Tzu, and Lhasa Apso) normally do not have scissors bites.

Malocclusion: Malocclusion refers to abnormal tooth alignment.

- **Overbite** (overshot, class two, overjet, mandibular brachygnathism)—occurs when the lower jaw is shorter than the upper. There is a gap between the upper and lower incisors when the mouth is closed. The upper premolars are displaced at least 25 percent toward the front when compared with the lower premolars.
- **Underbite** (undershot, reverse scissors bite, prognathism, class three)—occurs when the lower teeth protrude in front of the upper jaw teeth.
- **Even** or **level bite**—occurs when the upper and lower incisor teeth meet each other edge to edge.
- **Open bite**—occurs when the upper and lower incisors do not overlap or even meet each other when the mouth is closed.
- **Anterior crossbite**—occurs when the canine and premolar teeth on both sides of the mouth occlude normally but one or more of the lower incisors are positioned in front of the upper incisors. The anterior crossbite, the most common malocclusion, is not considered genetic or hereditary and is correctable.
- **Posterior crossbite**—occurs when one or more of the premolar lower jaw teeth overlap the upper jaw teeth. This rare condition occurs in the longer nosed dog breeds.
- **Wry bite**—occurs when one side of the jaw grows longer than the other. It is considered hereditary and difficult to correct.
- **Base narrow canines**—occur when the lower canine teeth protrude inward and can damage the upper palate. Often, this condition is due to retained baby teeth and can usually be corrected through inclined planes used to push the teeth into normal occlusion.

[Your letterhead here]

Feline Odontoclastic Resorptions and Stomatitis

The **feline odontoclastic resorptive lesion (FORL)** is a common feline dental problem. A majority of the cats affected are older than four years. These resorptions have also been called cavities, neck lesions, external or internal root resorptions, and cervical line erosions. FORLs are located usually where the gum line meets the tooth. The most common teeth affected are the lower third and first molars; however, FORLs can be found anywhere on any tooth. The cause is unknown.

Patients affected with FORLs may drool, bleed, or have difficulty eating. A majority of affected cats do not show clinical signs. Most times, it is up to the owner or veterinarian to diagnose the lesions on oral examination. Diagnostic aids include a periodontal probe or cotton-tipped applicator applied to the suspected FORL. The lesion often erodes into the sensitive dentin, causing the cat to show pain with jaw spasms when the FORL is touched.

FORLs can present in many stages:

Initially, in the **class one FORL, an enamel defect is noted**. The lesion is minimally sensitive because it has not entered dentin. Therapy for the defect usually involves thorough cleaning, polishing, and daily toothbrushing with a fluoride paste.

In **class two, lesions penetrate enamel and dentin**. Affected teeth may be treated with glass ionomer restoratives, which release fluoride ions to desensitize exposed dentin, strengthen enamel, and chemically bind to tooth surfaces. The long-term (greater than two years) effectiveness of restoration at this second stage of lesions has not been proven. Glass ionomer application to the FORL does not automatically stop the progression of the disease.

Radiographs are essential to determine if the lesions have **entered the pulp (class three)**, requiring either root canal therapy or extraction.

In the **class four FORL, the crown has been eroded or fractured**. Gum tissue grows over the root fragments, leaving a painful lesion that bleeds when probed. Treatment of choice is flap surgery and extraction of the root fragments when the tissue surrounding them appears inflamed or painful to the patient.

Cats can also be affected by **stomatitis**, a generalized inflammation of the mouth, called **lymphocytic plasmacytic gingivitis stomatitis (LPGS)**. The cause of this disease has not been determined. Affected cats will show signs including swallowing difficulty, weight loss, and drooling. When examining the mouth, you may see a cobblestone-appearing redness in the back of your cat's mouth. In addition, marked gingivitis and periodontitis exist around the premolars and molars.

Traditional therapy options include thorough cleaning and polishing, gum surgery, extraction, corticosteroids, gold therapy, Flagyl, megestrol acetate, and laser treatment.

Intraoral radiographs are taken of all the teeth. If a tooth is affected by moderate to severe periodontitis typified by greater than 50 percent bone loss, it should be extracted. In addition all root fragments need to be removed. Radiographs should be repeated after extraction to ensure complete tooth removal.

Immediately following surgery, prednisone is given daily and the dosage tapered over a three-week period. You will be advised how to brush your cat's teeth daily and to follow this with an irrigation of 2 percent chlorhexidine.

If the above therapy does not cure the disease within two months, or if the disease is severe, all teeth are removed behind the canines. Total mouth extractions will cure greater than 80 percent of the cats affected.

[Your letterhead here; a handout to be given to dental clients
when they arrive at your office]

What to Expect If Your Pet Needs Dental Care

Root canals, dental radiographs, orthodontics, crowns, caps, implants, and periodontal surgery for pets? You must be kidding! Not at all. Dental procedures are routinely performed in veterinary practices daily. How does a pet owner know if dental care is needed, and where can a pet owner go for advanced dental care?

Examination is the key to diagnosis and determination of the type of treatment needed. You need to know what to look for. You can help by examining your pet's teeth and oral cavity monthly. First smell the breath. If you note a disagreeable odor, gum disease may be present. Periodontal disease is the most common ailment of small animals. Gum problems begin when bacteria accumulate at the gum line around the tooth. Unless brushed away daily, bacteria will destroy tooth-supporting bone, cause bleeding, and, if untreated, result in tooth loss. Usually the first sign is bad breath. Other signs are red swollen gums, tartar (a yellow or brown accumulation on the tooth surface), and loose teeth.

When examining your pet's mouth, look for chips or fractures on the surface of the teeth. Contrary to their popularity, cow hooves, bones, or other hard materials chewed by pets may break teeth. Often, small pieces of enamel are chipped off, which causes no harm. Deeper chips into the dentin layer may cause sensitivity to your pet if not treated. If a fracture is deeper, you may notice a red, brown, or black spot in the middle of the tooth surface. The spot is the pulp (made up of the tooth's nerve and blood vessels), which is now open to oral cavity bacteria.

When your exam reveals dental problems, a trip to the veterinarian is in order. The veterinary oral examination will begin with visual examination of the face, mouth, and each tooth. Frequently, a pet's mouth has multiple problems that need care.

A detailed exam follows. Cats and dogs cannot point to dental abnormalities with their paws. In or-der to determine the proper treatment plan, other tests are necessary. Sedation and anesthesia are essential to adequately evaluate oral conditions. Anesthesia allows the veterinarian to examine each tooth individually and thoroughly.

Expect your veterinarian or dental assistant to use a periodontal probe to measure gum pocket depths around each tooth. One or 2 mm of probe depth normally exist around each tooth in the dog and 0.5 mm in the cat. When dogs or cats are affected by periodontal disease, depths increase, creating periodontal pockets. When the probe depth in cats and dogs is greater than 5 mm, periodontal disease is present, requiring additional care to save the tooth. Unfortunately, by the time some pets are presented for dental care, it is too late to save the teeth. Preventive care and periodic checkups help decrease the loss of additional teeth.

Radiographs show the inside of the tooth and root. Veterinarians use the same dental radiograph units that are used for humans. Many decisions are based on radiograph findings. Usually, the veterinarian will visually examine the mouth, note any problems, take radiographs while the animal is under anesthesia, and then tell you what needs to be done.

If your dog or cat needs advanced dental care, where can it be found? Many veterinarians have taken postgraduate dental training in order to better serve their patients. There are veterinarians who have passed advanced written and practical examinations given by the American Veterinary Medical Association, which certifies them as dental specialists. Veterinary dental specialists can consult with your veterinarian or see your dog or cat directly.

Dogs and cats do not have to suffer the pain and discomfort of untreated broken or loose teeth and infected gums. With the help of thorough examinations, radiographs, dental care, and daily brushing, your pet can keep its teeth in its mouth, where they should be.

[Your letterhead here; a handout to educate clients
about advanced periodontal care]

Consil—Savior for Some Hopeless Teeth

Periodontal disease is the most common of all small animal medical problems. Most dogs and cats over five years old will develop gum disease and bone loss around teeth. Unless you have been thoroughly brushing your pet's teeth daily from birth, this problem will affect your pet. Even so, you may ask why you should be concerned about a few loose teeth.

The area where the tooth meets the gum accumulates plaque daily. Plaque is an accumulation of bacteria. Unless teeth are brushed daily to remove plaque, mineral-rich calculus develops over plaque, which allows bacteria to reproduce under the gum line, causing infection and bone loss. Such infections often spread into the bloodstream and on to the kidneys and heart valves.

Unfortunately, bacterial by-products may destroy the tooth support, resulting in mobile teeth. In the past, loose teeth were extracted due to the body's inability to rebuild bone and ligament support. Now there is a way to save many of the teeth that were termed hopeless: Consil.

Consil is a synthetic bioactive ceramic material that bonds to bone as well as soft tissue and can even regenerate bone in periodontal pockets. It has been available as Bioglass for human periodontal care and has recently been approved for use in companion animals as Consil (Nutramax Laboratories, Baltimore, Maryland). The material is used to pack the bone loss area, it does not migrate from the surgical site, and it allows new bone and periodontal ligament to form. The veterinarian exposes the pocket via flap surgery, applies Consil, and sutures the site closed.

As with other periodontal procedures, daily tooth-brushing is advised. Thanks to Consil, many more dogs and cats will be able to keep their teeth and smiles.

[Your letterhead here]

Orthodontic Release

I understand that the orthodontic procedure to be performed on my pet is intended for the sole purpose of making the animal's bite comfortable and preventing the development of future dental disease.

The American Kennel Club (AKC) has rules against alterations of problems that are inherited.

I further understand that if the orthodontic problem is found to be genetically based, the animal will be removed from the breeding pool.

The procedure has been explained to me, and I fully understand the ethical and procedural parameters involved.

SIGNATURE OF THE OWNER _____

DATE _____

[Your letterhead here]

Referral Agreement

Your pet has been referred to us for dental consultation and treatment.

The veterinarian that sent you to us has confidence in our advanced training to care for your pet's dental needs. We wish to handle your pet's problem to the best of our ability and then send you back to your regular veterinarian for continued health care.

In this spirit of referral, please sign the statement below. By so signing, you agree not to ask us to care for any other problems your pet may have.

Thank you.

SIGNATURE OF THE OWNER _____

DATE _____

[Your letterhead here]

Home Care Instructions for Orthodontic Patients

Today, we installed an orthodontic corrective appliance in your pet's mouth. There are special instructions to ensure treatment success.

- Please check the mouth daily for movement or loss of the orthodontic appliance.

- Brush the teeth and orthodontic materials in the mouth with a soft-bristled toothbrush and animal toothpaste after each meal.

- Do not let your pet chew on hard objects such as toys, cow hooves, balls, pig's ears, or rawhide chews.

- Daily smell your pet's breath—a foul odor is an indication that your cleaning attempts are not sufficient. If the bad odor persists, please let us examine the mouth.

Your next visit is scheduled for: _____

Please do not feed your dog or cat at least 12 hours before the next visit because anesthesia may be necessary to replace or adjust the orthodontic appliance.

It is critical that the follow-up appointment schedule is adhered to.

[Your letterhead here]

Dental Anesthesia

Why does your pet have to be placed under anesthesia for dental care?

- Anesthesia keeps the pet immobile for examination and treatment.

- Anesthesia allows us to do what needs to be done in the shortest period of time without discomfort for the patient.

- Dental cleaning procedures require intubation (placing an endotracheal tube into the trachea) to prevent bacteria-laden debris from entering the respiratory system. This can only be done under general anesthesia.

How is anesthesia delivered? There are different ways to provide anesthesia, from intravenous or intramuscular sedation to general or inhaled routes. Each has its advantages and disadvantages.

- Intravenous anesthesia results in a fast induction (time from administration to the time the animal is asleep) but does not last long. Some intravenous anesthetics take longer to exit the body because they require metabolism by the liver and kidneys. In some cases sedation is sufficient to provide pain relief and motion control for short periods without having to use general anesthesia.

- Longer procedures (greater than 15 minutes) require general inhalant (gas) anesthesia. Gas is breathed in through a tube placed in the trachea and attached to an anesthetic machine, which mixes the vaporized anesthetic with oxygen. The degree of anesthesia (light, medium, and heavy) is controlled by the percentage of gas mixture. General anesthesia is delivered through the lungs. Most times after the procedure is finished, the dog or cat breathes off the anesthetic and recovers quickly.

We consider many factors such as age, the procedure to be performed, and preexisting conditions in order to choose the best anesthesia for the patient. Isoflurane is one of the newest and safest types of inhalation anesthetic used in small animal practice. In most cases a preanesthetic injection is given to sedate the patient, and then the gas is administered with a mask over the mouth. Once the pet is heavily sedated, an endotracheal tube is placed in the windpipe.

Safety is our most important concern. Before anesthetic delivery, the animal is examined, with particular attention given to heart and lung sounds. Diagnostic preoperative stool, urine, and blood testing of organ function are often performed to confirm that the patient can safely be anesthetized. We must be made aware of any preexisting medical conditions or medications your animal is taking.

The patient under anesthesia is constantly monitored. Observing the color of the gingiva and the number of respirations per minute are two ways. We use the electrocardiogram, respiratory monitor with apnea alarm, pulse oximeter (which measures the amount of oxygen inside the patient as well as the heart rate), and constant blood pressure monitor. These instruments add a level of safety to the procedure.

[Your letterhead here]

Disarming Waiver

Patient _____

Owner/agent _____

Disarming is a procedure used to reduce the height of canine teeth.

I have requested that the above named animal undergo this procedure. The procedure is used to make a potentially aggressive or vicious animal less dangerous by making the canine teeth dull and short.

I understand that animals that have had crown reduction may still be aggressive and vicious and that they may still bite people and other animals. I understand that crown reduction may reduce the severity of the injuries my animal may inflict but does not render a dangerous animal harmless. Every precaution must be taken when dealing with potentially dangerous animals to avoid situations that could lead to an attack.

I accept all liability for my animal's behavior and actions, including injury to people and animals.

SIGNATURE OF THE OWNER/AGENT _____

DATE _____

[Your letterhead here]

Twelve Steps of the Teeth-Cleaning/Diagnostic Visit

A dog or cat teeth cleaning means different things to different people. At our animal hospital the teeth-cleaning visit is a lot more than removing tartar from teeth. Our goal is to restore your pet's mouth to its normal, fresh, healthy state. Having your pet's teeth professionally cleaned is the single most important medical treatment you can give that will result in long-term health.

We are serious about keeping your pet's teeth as healthy as possible. Each teeth cleaning is performed at our hospital. There are 12 steps we take to ensure the best for your dog or cat.

What is involved in the teeth cleaning performed at our hospital?

1. A general exam before anesthesia, including evaluation of the bite, preoperative organ testing, and identification of abnormal wear patterns, gum infection, and oral cancer

2. An oral exam under anesthesia

3. Calculus removal from the visible part of the teeth

4. Subgingival (below-the-gum-line) scaling, root planing, and curettage where indicated. Removing tartar from the tooth crowns may improve the appearance of teeth, but dental disease is more proliferative below the gum line.

5. Tooth polishing

6. Irrigation of periodontal pockets with chlorhexidine solution

7. Fluoride application to create more resistant enamel and to reduce dental sensitivity

8. Postcleaning exam and radiographs if needed

9. Dental charting for the medical record

10. Therapy if necessary

11. Home care instructions on oral hygiene. Our dental technician will meet with you after the teeth cleaning to review toothbrushing techniques and your pet's custom-designed oral hygiene program, which is based on conditions found and your pet's willingness to be treated.

12. A no fee follow-up appointment and periodic rechecks to see how well you are performing home care

[A sample patient letter as a reminder to make an appointment
following periodontitis therapy; modify as needed]

Patient: Chelsea
Date of treatment: January 15, 1999
Diagnosis: Grade three periodontal disease

Dear Mrs. Brown:

On October 10, 1998, Chelsea was treated for periodontal disease.
As we discussed at that visit, her continued oral health requires home
care and frequent reexams. Her progress reexam is due now. The visit
consists of an oral exam without anesthesia in the exam room to evaluate healing and oral home care effectiveness. We will also review brushing techniques to help you get to those areas where tartar may be accumulating.

The exam will also allow us to see if additional therapy is needed.
Periodontal disease is progressive and if untreated may result in pain
plus the spread of infection to other areas of the body. Chelsea depends
on your cooperation.

Please call our office for an appointment for this evaluation. There
will not be a fee for the exam other than that for anesthesia and
additional therapy if necessary. If you have any questions, call to speak
to Brandi, our dental technician, or myself.

Sincerely,

Jan Bellows, DVM
DIPLOMATE, AMERICAN VETERINARY DENTAL COLLEGE

[A sample patient letter as a reminder to make an appointment
following gingivitis therapy; modify as needed]

Patient: Chelsea
Date of treatment: January 15, 1999
Diagnosis: Grade one gingivitis

On October 10, we examined Chelsea and professionally cleaned, scaled, and polished her teeth. To help promote optimal dental health, we recommend periodic reexams. That time is now upon us.

During this visit we will evaluate how successful home care and regular toothbrushing have been. We will also review brushing techniques should there be any problem areas where tartar is still accumulating. If in fact there is any tartar buildup, we will recommend that the teeth be professionally cleaned.

When plaque accumulates at the gum line of dogs and cats, inflammation, infection, gingivitis, and eventually periodontal disease can result. Periodontitis is irreversible and if left untreated can result in pain or, worse yet, the spread of infection to other parts of the body. Our goal is to work with you to prevent this and to keep Chelsea's teeth and gums healthy and free of disease.

Please call our office at your earliest convenience to schedule an appointment. There will be no fee for this exam; however, if cleaning is necessary, the usual fees will of course be applicable. Should you require any additional information, please feel free to call us. If for whatever reason I am unavailable, our dental technician Brandi will be happy to answer your questions.

Hope to see you soon.

Sincerely yours,

Jan Bellows, DVM
DIPLOMATE, AMERICAN VETERINARY DENTAL COLLEGE

Appendix 2
❧SOURCES OF DENTAL EQUIPMENT AND INFORMATION

COMPANY	PRODUCT	PHONE NUMBER
Addison Biological Laboratory, Inc.	Maxiguard	660-248-2215
AFP Imaging Corporation	DentX Radiograph Unit	800-592-6666, ext. 403
American Society of Veterinary Dental Technicians (ASVDT)	Veterinary dental technician organization and training	800-613-3647
Cbi (Charles Brungart, Inc.)	Scalers, high-speed delivery system	800-654-5705
Cislak Manufacturing, Inc.	Dental hand instruments	800-239-2904
CK Dental Specialties	Endodontic equipment and hand instruments	800-675-CKDS
DentaLabel Company	Adhesive dental charts	800-662-7920
Gel Kam International (Colgate Oral Pharmaceuticals)	Stannous fluoride gel	800-527-0222
Henry Schein, Inc.	Full line of human and veterinary dental supplies	800-272-4346
Heska	Perioceutic and home care products	800-GO-HESKA
Hill's Pet Nutrition, Inc.	Tartar control diet	800-354-4557
Hu-Friedy Company	Hand instruments	800-729-3743
Lester A. Dine, Inc.	Dental camera/imaging	800-624-9103
Luxar	CO_2 laser	800-548-1482
Microcopy	Radiograph processing fluids	800-235-1863
Med Rx, Inc.	Vetscope	888-392-1234
Nylabone Products	Home care chewing aids	800-631-2188
Omni Products International	Fluoride gel	800-284-4123
Orascoptic Research	Illuminated telescopes	800-369-3698
Pharmacia & Upjohn Animal Health	Dental antibiotic, dental models, and dental educational materials	800-253-8600
Precision Ceramics Dental Lab	Crowns, orthodontic appliances	800-223-6322
Sage-London Industries	Dental power and hand instruments	800-461-9383
Tulsa Dental Products	Endodontic files and equipment	800-662-1202
Virbac	Home care products	800-338-3659
VRX Pharmaceuticals	Full line of oral care products	800-969-7387

❧INDEX